CHIROPRACTIC
HEALTH
CENTER

coyote

Dr. Daniel Piper, Chiropractic Physician

4124 Quebec Ave. N. #307 • New Hope, MN 55427
Office 612-533-9819 • Fax 612-533-0961

AN APPLE
A DAY?

Is It
Enough
Today?

═══════════════════════

Dr. M. Ted Morter, Jr.

BEST RESEARCH, INC.

An Apple A Day?: Is It Enough Today?

Dr. M. Ted Morter, Jr.

Copyright © 1996, B.E.S.T. Research, Inc.

Printed in the United States
ISBN 0-944994-07-5

Morter HealthSystem
1000 West Poplar Street
Rogers, Arkansas 72756

1 800 874 1478
1 501 631 8201 (Fax)

*Dedicated to all those who want to
improve their quality of life.*

INFORMATION FOR THE READER

TABLE OF CONTENTS

INTRODUCTION

SURVIVING NUTRITION

Cut down on dietary fat for healthy heart and arteries. Take an aspirin a day to reduce the risks of cancer and/or heart attacks. Exercise regularly for fitness. As the years roll on, have high-tech tests done to see if you're headed for serious or life-threatening disease. Avoid stress — adjust your attitude and think relaxing, positive thoughts. Don't smoke cigarettes or hang around those who do. Then after you've done all that and followed other bits of advice too numerous to mention, see your doctor to find out what's gone wrong.

There's something not-quite-right about this scenario.

If you're doing everything right, why do things go wrong?

Actually, things inside your body don't "go wrong." As long as they go at all, they're going right — for the circumstances.

You see, you were designed to survive. You weren't designed to be healthy or sick. Your body adapts its physiology — its internal workings — to suit every stimulus, or signal, it receives. It responds to signals that come to it from the outside through your five senses — loud noises, familiar holiday aromas, flashing blue lights, compliments, insults, good food, bad food, pure water, treated water, prescription drugs, illegal drugs, clean air, polluted air, gory action flicks, love stories, whatever. And it responds to signals generated from the inside — your internal monitoring systems, thoughts, memories, and emotions. Whether the signals come from the outside or inside, your body will respond to keep itself alive! This signal-response ballet is directed solely for the purpose of survival right now.

The results of all of the survival responses put together are what we call health or pain and sickness — ease or dis-ease.

Your body doesn't care if you are sick or healthy. It doesn't plan for the future. Your body doesn't think and it doesn't judge. It doesn't care if you're hurting or happy. All it does is respond to survive. Your body makes thousands of perfect survival responses every instant of your life. You may like the results of the responses and call it "health." Or you may not like the results and call it "disease." Your body doesn't care whether you like the results or not. What a bummer!

WELLNESS PRINCIPLE: You do health or disease; your body does survival.

You create health or disease opportunities when you act on your personal choices of what you put into or do to your body. Your body responds to everything you do, think, and feel. It has no choice. It doesn't choose to respond or not respond. And it doesn't choose how it will respond. It's all automatic.

Health and disease are both effects. Each is the effect of accumulated physiological survival responses. When you eat, drink, breathe, exercise, rest, and think, some part of your body's physiology changes. You constantly make conscious choices about these six activities. Keep making the same choices over and over and your body responds the same way over and over. Whatever your body does is perfect for whatever caused the response. If the responses lead to health, great. If responses lead to disease, that's great, too — you're alive. Your body is still able to respond.

That's what health, either good or not-so-good, is about — whole-body survival responses to everything you do. And you consciously control most of the things your body must survive in order to get "health" results rather than "disease" results.

WELLNESS PRINCIPLE: Health and disease are twins.

Survival responses are always perfect. Response control is the job of your subconscious. You have little conscious control over internal responses. You do have conscious control over most of the signals that spark the responses. It's the signals you can control that are the real bottom-line *cause* of disease. This book is one of a series written specifically to help you understand that you can control many situations that produce response signals your body must survive.

Why a series? Because you have conscious control over choices you make in three basic areas of life: (1) what you put into your body — what you eat and drink; (2) what you do with and to your body — how you exercise, rest, and breathe, and; (3) what you say to yourself in your internal conversations — what you think and feel about yourself and your life. Your body responds to signals from these choice activities all the time. To keep you alive, it must survive all of these activities. Your body doesn't need your help to carry out its survival functions. Your body needs for you to make choices that don't interfere with it doing its job.

We begin the series with *An Apple A Day?* — the "what you eat and drink" choices we call "diet." Eating and drinking are nice, tangible, easy-to-monitor activities. Many people see diet as the cornerstone of health. Yet, as you will see, diet is just one layer of the cornerstone of health. Exercise, rest, breathing, and thinking are the other layers of your health cornerstone. In other books, you will also see how diet and exercise can team up to make you fit, or make you dead. And, most important, you will see why your thoughts and feelings about yourself, the things you've done, and the things that have been done to you are the most potent body-response generators of all.

This book deals with how your body responds to the substances you put into it. It's not about fat, calories, cholesterol, or the latest vitamin or mineral craze. It's about giving your body the kinds of foods that determine if the "climate" of your internal environment is "healthy" — the kinds that allow your systems, organs, and cells to survive without undue stress. When your internal environment is healthy, your cells are healthy. When your cells are healthy, your organs and systems are healthy. And when your organs and systems are healthy, you are healthy. Simple as that!

The objective of this book is to help you to understand that the body is *alkaline by design and acid by function*™. Your internal fluids are designed to be slightly alkaline. Yet, when your cells work, which they do all the time, they produce internal acid. However, that's part of the design. Your body is designed to eliminate this acid very easily. On the other hand, foods such as meat, poultry, fish, grains, and nuts bring with them a type of acid that is not as easily eliminated. When there's too much acid in the body, the internal environment is "polluted." Systems, organs, and cells can't work at their best.

WELLNESS PRINCIPLE: **Your body is** *alkaline by design and acid by function.*

But you're not doomed to having a lot of dietary acid sloshing around your internal environment and causing trouble. Remember those immortal words that reverberated through your childhood: "Eat your vegetables!" Fruits and vegetables bring with them vital minerals your body uses to take care of the strong acid left by the meats, poultry, fish, and grains. These minerals are a vital part of the survival plan.

The recurring theme throughout this book is that the body is designed to survive immediate problems. It does whatever is necessary to clean up its internal environment. If the same "immediate situation" continues over time, organs and systems are overworked. Overworked organs and systems become exhausted and symptoms appear. The symptoms are then named osteoporosis, multiple sclerosis, Parkinson's disease, heart attack, or whatnot.

This is not an abstinence, never-eat-meat-or-other-things-you-like book. It is about balance. You'll find that your body can handle not-best-for-survival foods occasionally. You'll also find out why some foods raise your acid potential, and how ingredients in vegetables and fruits neutralize acid to keep your internal environment at its best. And you'll get some pointers on menus that will help turn healthy eating into a pleasure.

WELLNESS PRINCIPLE: Healthy eating is not a penance.

There must be a better path to health, happiness, and success than the one we're on — and there is. Health, happiness, and success are by-products of personal decisions. Health, happiness, and success are the result of making more right decisions than wrong. Health is the result of making more right decisions than wrong about eating, drinking, exercising, resting, breathing, and thinking. These decision areas affect your whole body all the time. So instead of trying to figure out what to do to pamper each organ or function of your body, how about making sure that you're giving your whole body the opportunity to be healthy?

That's what this series is about. Recognizing opportunities to improve overall and all-over health. And once recognized, taking personal responsibility to improve your chances of living a more healthful, satisfying life. Best of all, the methods outlined in this series don't put a crimp in the pocketbook. In fact, they don't cost anything other than time and commitment. Here's to your healthy, happy, successful future.

CHAPTER 1

PREVIEW OF COMING ATTRACTIONS

OVERVIEW

Health gurus preach it. The medical profession advises it. And, now, even the government recommends it. "Eat more veggies and less red meat." Everyone seems to be taking up the chant. The reason for this major change in dietary recommendations isn't clearly defined by the health care sages. The implication is that those who eat lots of vegetables and fruit seem to be healthier, have fewer aches and pains, and possibly live longer than those who eat lots of meat. But, so far, "they" haven't told us "why."

You're about to find out "why." You'll learn why and how the *types* of foods you eat can affect your long-term health. And to help you put the concepts into practice, you'll find menus that are part of *The Feelin' Good Program.* This program is a guide to eating better to feel better. But more about that later in the book.

Between these covers, you'll find a view of food-health that's a little different from the view usually held in our society. The health factor in foods is *the effect on your internal environment* of remnants of digested food. It's not just artery-clogging fatty foods or chocked-full-of-cholesterol foods. It's not just calorie-laden starchy foods or nutrient-sparse fast foods that are behind many of our health woes. It's a whole body too-much-acid problem.

As a sneak preview, I'll tell you that high-protein foods are the major strong acid offenders. And too much dietary acid from protein (or anything else) isn't good. Fruits and vegetables, although acid themselves, for the most part, don't leave strong acid. We'll go into that later, too.

To put the part about food and food types in perspective, we'll first look at why your diet is just one feature of your life that affects your health. Your body *functions* as a whole, complete unit, and it *survives* as a whole, complete unit. Everything you do affects your whole body, and thinking is one of the things you do all the time.

WELLNESS PRINCIPLE: You are more than a collection of parts.

THE WHOLE YOU

You are much more than an assortment of parts packed neatly within your visible skin. You developed as a complete unit and you continue to function as a complete unit. Anything and everything that affects one part of you affects the whole you. When you jog or exert yourself, your heart, lungs, muscles, circulation, blood acid level, digestive processes, and bunches of other internal organs and processes are affected. When you are upset, your heart, lungs, muscles, circulation, blood acid level, digestive processes, and bunches of other internal organs and processes are affected. No matter what you do, all functions of your body are directly or indirectly involved.

The main thing to understand is that you are a unified being. You aren't like your minivan, TV, or lawn mower. You weren't made up of component parts and assembled for delivery.

WELLNESS PRINCIPLE: **You are a synchronized, harmonious, interacting whole.**

Pain and disease in any part of the whole are effects of a "whole" problem. Pain and disease in themselves aren't the problem. They just hurt or kill. You aren't sick because your joints, head, or stomach hurt. You aren't sick because you have chronic fatigue syndrome, fibromyalgia, or Crohn's disease. These are merely names for particular symptoms. Symptoms are effects of the way particular systems, organs, or tissues are adapting to survive. Symptoms aren't the cause of your problem. You were sick before the symptoms showed up. A particular complaint is merely the way sickness shows itself in a particular body. In other words, health and disease are both side-effects of the responses your body has made to the conditions it must survive. And for the most part, the conditions it must survive are brought about by decisions or choices you have made over time in six essential areas of life.

DECIDEDLY HEALTHY

Every day of your conscious existence you make decisions. Conscious choices. Some decisions affect your future more than others. Your decision to change your job can alter your life. Yet, your decision to have the paper towels come off the top of the roll rather than the bottom doesn't make even a tiny day-altering ripple.

However, other seemingly inconsequential decisions you make every day can affect your future as much as job decisions. Every day you decide how you will respond in six vital areas of life. You decide what you eat and drink, what you think, what you breathe, and how you exercise and rest. Each of the six decision areas is so important to your current health and well-being that I call the group *The Six Essentials of Life*. This book deals with the "eat" and "drink" essentials.

Choices in the six essentials are so common-place that most people don't even recognize them as conscious decisions. Eat and drink decisions are often based on ease, speed, and convenience. Exercise and rest choices are usually based on schedule loads. Choices you make in the six essentials usually aren't dramatic; they're constant.

> **WELLNESS PRINCIPLE:** The six essentials are requirements of living.

You can't survive without any one of the six essentials for very long. If you do, you set up a crisis situation for your body. And "very long" differs for each essential area. You can go without eating, drinking, exercising, and resting a lot longer than you can go without breathing. And, as long as you are conscious, you think — whether you like it or not.

The fallout from your choices in the six essential areas affects how you feel and how healthy you are. When the decisions you make in all six areas keep your body functioning at its best, you are healthy and you feel good. If you consistently make essential decisions that keep your body in crisis, you are — or will be — sick. That's not an over statement; it's just the way things are.

Although diet is the most popular area of an I'm-going-to-improve-my-life campaign, thoughts and feelings are the most important areas. Your body responds constantly and intensely to how you feel about everything that goes on in your life. And these responses can be behind major physical problems. But it will take another whole book to go into that.

SURVIVAL FIRST

Survival of this instant is your body's only goal. Not survival later today, or next week, or next year. Survival now. Your body was designed to survive. It wasn't designed to be sick. It wasn't designed to be healthy. And it has done its survival job very well, or you wouldn't be reading these words now.

You may not be happy with the by-products of your body's survival techniques. You may have aches and pains that range from annoying to excruciating. You may be in the throes of a serious disease. Or you may be in the process of developing a disease that you haven't even noticed yet because you are still symptom free. No matter where you register on your

personal health scale — anywhere between really
healthy and really sick — your body is doing exactly
what it was designed to do to survive. It is surviving
the conditions imposed on it. For instance . . .

Those who are constantly anxious, afraid, up-
tight, jealous, judgmental, or self-critical (which
certainly doesn't include you), keep their bodies ready
for a fight. Being ready for a fight is fine if they're in
physical danger. But being ready for a fight
constantly — days, nights, and weekends — is really
hard on the old bod'. After a while, it gets exhausted.
And you know what happens when *you* get exhausted
— your performance suffers. Well, your body works
the same way. The difference is that your body's
performance is perfect — for exhausted conditions.
The perfect performance may not lead to pain-free
health, but it's perfect for surviving exhausting
conditions. If the exhaustion continues, organs and
systems curtail production or shut down.

WELLNESS PRINCIPLE: **No system or organ can
function with the pedal to the
metal all the time without
breaking down.**

Usually, the first organs or systems to go are
those that aren't contributing to *immediate* survival.
For example, you can manage with gallstones a lot
better than you can manage with acidic blood. You
can get along better without a full complement of
calcium in your bones than you can without strong
heart muscle contractions. And you certainly don't
need to be digesting food when you're defending
against an aggressive grizzly.

The good news is that you have control over most of the situations your body must survive. Well, maybe not the grizzly. However, the choices you make in the six essentials set up the survival threats your body must respond to. And the biggest survival threat is stress.

SURVIVING STRESS

Stress is a change in environment that prompts a response. All mental and physical activities *stress* your body. *Stress is anything that causes your body to change the way it is functioning right now.* Remember that. It's important.

> **WELLNESS PRINCIPLE:** **Anything that causes your body to change what it is doing right now is a stress to your body.**

Your life may be stress city. You may get bent out of shape over a variety of stresses — job trauma, traffic snarls, weird-family syndrome, overactive or underactive household plumbing, dwindling dollars, frazzled relationships, and the like. But your body contends with only three types of stress: physical, mental, and nutritional.

Physical stress comes from outside your body. It's the charging grizzly, a fall down the stairs, a cut or burn, or anything that you interpret as a potential threat to life and limb. Your response to physical threat is quick, automatic, and without much thought. You get out of the way or you stand your ground and fight. You recognize the physical stress,

you respond, and in a short time, both stress and
response are over. Survival at its best.

Physical stress also includes exercise. Whether it's
turning the pages of a book, raking leaves, walking,
jogging, or running like crazy from a gallumping
Doberman, it's physical stress your body is designed
to handle with ease. After the incident is over, the
stress is gone.

WELLNESS PRINCIPLE: **Physical stresses are short-
term stresses.**

Mental stress comes from inside your body — your
mental interpretations of the world around you. This
is the stress you generate yourself when you hang
onto feelings of worry, anxiety, jealousy, fear, guilt, or
any of the other negative emotions. There's no actual
physical threat that you can confront and resolve.
And, usually, there's no closure to the incident.

WELLNESS PRINCIPLE: **Mental stress is long-term
and devastating to your body.**

Nutritional stress can be short-term or long-term.
Short-term nutritional stress comes every time you
eat or drink something. Put food into your mouth and
your body immediately changes what it is doing. It
handles the situation, then goes back to business as
usual. Each meal or snack is a short-term stress.
Long-term nutritional stress comes from eating the
wrong types of foods for months, years, or a lifetime.
The chapters that follow explain how some types of
foods contribute to long-term nutritional stress.

WELLNESS PRINCIPLE: **Long-term nutritional stress can be a major cause of serious degenerative diseases.**

The objective of this series is to help you recognize how your choices in the six essential areas of life may be inflicting long-term stresses on your body. Again, short-term stress usually comes from the outside as a threat to your physical well-being — the screech of a smoke alarm in the night, an attention-getting thump on the shin from running into the open door of a dishwasher, the earth-shaking rumble of a rhino charging at you from the brush, or other threatening experience. Short-term stress is quick, on and off, "hit and run" stress.

Long-term stress is the disease-producer. Long-term stress comes from the inside: mental, emotional, and nutritional stress — mental and emotional stress from thoughts and attitudes that keep your body up-tight, and nutritional stress from eating *too much* high-protein food.

Mental, emotional, and nutritional stresses exhaust both you and your internal organs and systems. Exhaustion leads to disease. When you reduce or eliminate long-term mental, emotional, and nutritional stress, you reduce or eliminate the need for your systems and organs to work overtime. You protect them from becoming exhausted. Eventually, like after 90 or 110 years, systems and organs may wear out. None of us will last forever, even under the best circumstances. However, when your body responds primarily to short-term physical stresses, health — not disease — becomes necessary.

WELLNESS PRINCIPLE: Your body doesn't do reality checks on stress.

Stress comes in many forms. Drink a glass of the purest water in the world, eat a poisonous mushroom, fall out of an airplane, sprint for the bus, celebrate your favorite team's victory, or clench your fists in frustration, and your body must respond to the new condition. If you are threatened, your body *must* respond. If you *think* you are being threatened, your body *must* respond. And since your body's sole purpose is to survive, it will respond perfectly to survive each and every threat.

WELLNESS PRINCIPLE: Every response your body makes is perfect!

PERFECT RESPONSES

The concept that every response of the body is perfect may be new to you. But think about it for a moment. Your body was designed to survive. Every response your body makes is directed toward surviving conditions of the moment. Everything it does is perfect for survival. Your body can't do anything wrong. In order to do something wrong, it would have to do something it wasn't designed to do. But it can't do that. Your body never — repeat, Never! — makes a mistake in the way it responds to any stimulus.

"C'mon," you might think, "if the body never makes a mistake, how come I have high blood pressure, my sister has arthritis, my father has diabetes, and millions of people die of heart disease?

Obviously, these bodies must be doing something wrong."

It would certainly seem so, according to our present perspective of health. We have been conditioned to believe that when we're sick, the body is running amuck. So what do we do? First, we itemize the symptoms and give them a name. Now we have a "disease" to treat. So we drug, radiate, or cut. We go after the "disease." The war on cancer. Searching for a cure for the common cold. Telethons, radiothons, walk-a-thons. All sorts of "-thons" are held to raise money to help "stamp out" all sorts of diseases. And that's good. People suffering from these diseases benefit, and researchers exploring the diseases benefit.

However, treating disease or symptoms seldom (if ever) gets to the *cause* of the problem. Symptoms are effects. Symptoms lumped together under a disease name are still effects — effects of the body responding perfectly to survive the stimuli it receives. When you treat disease, you treat effects of those responses. When you change or remove the stimuli that prompted the response, you address the cause. Disease becomes unnecessary.

WELLNESS PRINCIPLE: **If you don't like the response, change the stimulus.**

Of course, I am not saying, nor am I implying, that you should not treat disease or symptoms. I am saying that in a truly healthy body, disease is unnecessary. However, if you are having a heart attack, a severe asthma attack, or any other severe physical condition, that's the time to take care of the crisis. That's not the time to try to make disease unnecessary. You make disease unnecessary either before or after a physical crisis by controlling stimuli that can exhaust your body and lead to disease. If you take control before you are in physical trouble, you are in better shape to avoid the problem. When you control the stimuli — food, thoughts, breathing, and so forth — you address the cause of disease, not the effects.

WELLNESS PRINCIPLE: Don't just keep mopping up the water; fix the leak.

The decisions you make about foods help to determine the internal climate of your body. The major part of being healthy is keeping your cells healthy and their environment hospitable. That's the food factor — keeping your internal climate a neat place for cells to live and thrive. But just eating right doesn't assure health. Eating only foods that are good for you isn't the be-all-end-all of health.

The decisions you make about everyday activities — what you eat, drink, think and do — affect the climate of your cells' home and the way your body works. When you make and carry out decisions that allow a favorable internal climate, health is your reward. On the other hand, when you make and carry out decisions that produce an internal climate in which your body must constantly "fight for its life," pain and disease are your rewards.

WELLNESS PRINCIPLE: The choices you make determine your level of health, happiness, and success.

So this series is about how and why the decisions you make in the six essential areas of life determine how your body functions. Your essential decisions determine whether you are energetic, pain-free, and vibrantly alive, or you are always tired, hurting, and barely coping with life. This series explains why and how your body responds to and survives the things you do to it, and the things you put into it. Health and disease are by-products of how your body functions.

In the pages that follow we'll look at how your decisions concerning the types of foods and beverages you consume affect your body as a whole. In the books that follow, we'll look at how your decisions concerning thoughts, exercise, rest, and breathing affect your body as a whole. So let's get on with it. The best is yet to come.

CHAPTER 2

THE ACID FACTOR

HEALTH — FABLE AND FACT

Count your fat grams. Check your cholesterol. Watch your calories. Easy on the salt. Use margarine instead of butter. Use butter instead of margarine. Olive oil may help prevent breast cancer — and then again, it may not. Get plenty of Vitamin LPC (Latest Popular Craze).

You get the picture. Live-longer-feel-better advice changes about as often as you change your socks. How are we to sort fable from fact?

By injecting a little common sense into the ongoing eating-for-health binge. No single food, or vitamin, or mineral, or enzyme, or combination of foods will guarantee health or guard against disease. There is no "magic bullet" for health. Just eating right doesn't assure health. Exercising regularly doesn't assure health. Taking vitamin tablets, aspirin, shark cartilage, or powered gnats' tongues doesn't assure you'll be healthy. Health isn't static. Your body isn't static. They're both dynamic. Health changes

according to the levels, types, and duration of stress
your body must adapt to.

WELLNESS PRINCIPLE: Health is a process.

Health and disease are shorthand terms for how
your body is responding to everything you do and eat.
The term "healthy" usually means, "I don't hurt
much, am reasonably energetic, and can function
reasonably well." We usually use the term "disease"
to mean, "I hurt, don't have much energy, and can't
move as well as I would like."

The full-scope of the body's workings are complex
beyond our present understanding. No one knows all
about everything that influences the constant
internal chemical and electrical responses that keep
the body going. But my clinical experience indicates
that the choices you make in the six essentials set
you up for health, happiness, and success, or for
disease, misery, and failure.

**WELLNESS PRINCIPLE: Health comes from doing
most things right most of the
time.**

HEALTH IS AN INSIDE JOB

My thirty-plus years of clinical experience show
that your "internal environment" — the
"climate" in which your cells live — is the biggest
factor in how your body functions. Your body hums
along easily when it has the proper "tools" to work
with and when it doesn't need to stumble through
unnecessary junk to get to those tools.

That's not too surprising. Most of us work the same way. In pleasant surroundings, we accomplish greater and better things, are more at ease, and life goes more smoothly than in messy surroundings. Working in a clean, neat, uncontaminated environment with proper tools and equipment makes any job easier and less exhausting.

What does that have to do with food?

Back to your internal environment. The foods you put into your body help determine the environment in which your cells live. Your diet and drink choices can make your internal environment less than the best for your cells, organs, and systems.

When your cells live in an atmosphere that is best for them, they work better, longer, and manage day-to-day stress without being worn to a frazzle. When your internal environment is a mess, cells and systems must work harder to clean up the mess so your body can survive. That's exhausting. And you know where exhaustion leads — pain, disease, and all sorts of places you don't want to go.

I can't help you clean up messes outside your body. But I can help you to understand which kinds of foods make an internal mess.

MESSY FOODS

High-protein foods are messy foods. High-protein foods are foods such as hamburgers, chicken nuggets, smoked turkey breast, catfish, shrimp, and any other food that comes from formerly live, move-about creatures. High-protein foods also include goodies such as peanut butter, pinto beans, spaghetti, and pizza. The biggest internal mess your body must clean up is the leftovers of digested high-protein foods.

There's nothing wrong with high-protein foods themselves. The problem is with eating too much of them for too many years. After a while, your internal environment is a real mess. And the mess comes from *acid*.

When you eat a lot of high protein foods, your stomach produces strong acid to digest it. That's good. But the protein itself leaves acid that takes a scenic tour of your body. There's acid all over the place — where it should be and where it shouldn't be. That's not good.

The fluid in your stomach should be acid. The fluid in the rest of your body — blood, lymph, gallbladder bile, pancreatic fluid, saliva — shouldn't. None of those fluids should be the least little bit acid. However, if you eat too much protein for too long, internal fluids and life-support systems become too acid. That means your cells live in a mess.

WELLNESS PRINCIPLE: **Too much dietary protein pollutes your internal environment.**

BUT WE NEED PROTEIN

Right! We need protein. Protein is a major building block of cells. Cells are the building blocks of us. In cells, there's more protein than any other substance except water. When you consider that each of us is made up of about 75 trillion cells, that's a lot of protein and water.

We can't live without protein any better than we can live without water. And, as you will see, just about everything you eat has protein in it. Even fruits and vegetables!

Proteins are everywhere in your body. They come in a variety of forms. They perform a variety of functions. Proteins are good stuff. They are a source of heat and energy. They are essential for growth, for building new tissue, and for repairing damaged tissue. Your hair is mostly protein. The mechanisms that cause your muscles to contract are protein. Protein is inside the cells (*intracellular*), and outside the cells (*extracellular*).

WELLNESS PRINCIPLE: Different kinds of protein perform different jobs.

Some proteins are mainly *enzymes*. Enzymes spark chemical reactions when they come in contact with other substances in the cell. Enzymes control cellular *metabolism* — chemical energy changes within your cells.

Other proteins are *nucleoproteins* that contain DNA (deoxyribonucleic acid). Anyone who has watched TV in the past year or so is familiar with the term "DNA." DNA is made up of genes that pass hereditary characteristics — eye, hair, and skin color, body height and build, early baldness, nose shape, ear size, freckles, and much more — from your forefathers and foremothers to you and your children. DNA also controls the overall function of cells.

WELLNESS PRINCIPLE: You can't do without the proteins within.

So we have the protein paradox: Protein is a vital ingredient in your body. Your body can't do without protein. And you need protein in your diet. However, eating *too much* protein is behind many of our physical problems. Why? It's all . . .

A MATTER OF LEFTOVERS

Your body's internal environment is affected both by what you eat and by what's left over in your internal system after what you've eaten has been digested. Most foods leave post-digestion leftovers. Foods such as hamburgers, broccoli, ice cream, pizza, peanuts, or grapes leave an "after-glow" called *ash*. A few foods, such as refined sugar, honey, and corn syrup leave little, if any, ash.

"Ash? Inside my body?" you ask incredulously.

Indeed. Ash is the leftovers of "oxidized food fuel." The ash in your body is similar to the ash left from logs — the fuel — burned in your fireplace. But since internal ash is in a fluid environment, the ash isn't dry. It isn't stacked in neat little fluffy piles. However, it can "blow" around your body anyway. It didn't result from dancing flames. It's the part your body can't "burn" to produce energy — it's incombustible.

Ash is the part of food that's left after your body has used the good stuff — vitamins, minerals, enzymes. Ash is part of the useless stuff that must be eliminated — roughage and other undigested food remnants.

> **WELLNESS PRINCIPLE:** **Ash is the leftovers from "internal combustion."**

Ash from foods comes in essentially two "flavors" — acid and alkaline. The ash of high-protein foods is a fairly strong acid. Strong acid burns. The ash of most vegetables and fruit is the opposite of acid, it's alkaline. Very strong alkali can burn, too. But slight alkalinity, the strength best for your body, is soothing. For now, think of acid as being like vinegar — harsh and burny, and think of alkaline as being like bicarbonate of soda, or baking soda — mild and soothing.

WELLNESS PRINCIPLE: Vinegar is acid; baking soda is alkaline.

Your body must handle ash leftovers as best it can. Most fruit, including citrus fruits, and most vegetables leave alkaline leftovers — minerals that can assist in handling dietary acid. Foods that leave alkaline ash are called "alkaline ash-producing" foods. Remember, it's the leftovers we're talking about. The foods themselves aren't necessarily alkaline. You might think that lemons or grapefruit would be strong acid producers. Actually, even though lemons and grapefruit themselves are very acid in their natural state, they leave an alkaline ash, not acid ash. It's meats, grains, and most nuts that leave acid ash. We call these "acid ash-producing" foods. The ash of acid ash-producing foods contains fairly strong acid, especially for inside your body.

Your body was designed to handle little skirmishes with an occasional invasion of acid ash-producing foods. The acid can be eliminated. But first, it must be *neutralized* — toned down, buffered, made weaker.

No problem. You come equipped with neutralizing minerals that take care of the situation nicely. These minerals are part of your *alkaline reserve*. And as long as you don't abuse your neutralizing system, your internal environment chugs along rather smoothly. That's the way you were designed.

The crunch comes if you abuse the system. Every time you eat foods that leave an acid ash that must be neutralized, you lose precious minerals. That's no big deal for a six-year-old who still has a generous neutralizing mineral supply. But, munch mostly acid ash-producing foods at meals and snacks, day-after-day, month-after-month and eventually the built-in supply of neutralizing minerals will fall to crisis level. You have an internal emergency. Even our hypothetical six-year-old can be headed toward an internal emergency in a few years. But, who would relate a serious illness in an eleven- or twelve-year-old with all of those hot dogs and soft drinks he had lived on since his first tooth appeared?

But the body was designed to survive. So what does it do when its standard store of neutralizing minerals runs low?

It handles the emergency by finding other neutralizing minerals from around the body to do the job. It calls on its "special forces" — the internal equivalent of Green Berets, SEALS, and SWAT teams. If your neutralizing mineral supply is low, too much strong acid is an even more serious threat to survival. When you eat too much high-protein, acid ash-producing food, more strong acid is left than your body can handle without calling on backups.

Sounds like a perfect solution, doesn't it? Your body knows how to survive and will use all of the resources available to make sure it does as long as possible. As long as there are backups, all is well — right?

Not quite right.

Backup systems are short-term, handle-the-crisis systems. They're not meant to handle day-to-day operations. Backup systems are like your local fire department — available for emergencies. Always on call. Always ready to handle emergencies. Take care of the situation, get things out of crisis mode and back on an even keel, then rest until the next emergency. Backup systems, like fire fighters, should be temporary help only.

WELLNESS PRINCIPLE: **Backup systems and emergency crews need rest between crises.**

TELL TALE SIGNS

Your survival oriented body comes equipped with many backup systems. And there are backup systems for the backup systems. It's a beautiful design. Yet, despite our wealth of internal backup systems, most of us slog through our days with much more acid sloshing in our bodies than is good for us. Too much acid. Excess acidity. Acidosis. Our bodies are *toxic* — they are being "poisoned" by too much acid. But since we don't come with a built-in, solid-state, digital LED display acid meter, how do we know?

One way to tell is with pH test paper — litmus type paper.

You remember litmus paper from your high school chemistry days. Stick a specially treated narrow strip of paper into a solution. If the paper turns red, the solution is acid; if it stays blue, the solution is alkaline. You can use pH test paper to give you an idea of the overall acid-alkaline level of your body.

No, you don't stab your finger, draw blood and dip the paper in it. You check your urine.

"Check my urine???? You've got to be kidding!!!"

Nope. Think of it as detective work — like rummaging through a victim's trash to find clues to solve a mystery. But this is neater. Your urine contains many of your body's discards. You can learn a lot from the things your body throws away.

But you don't rummage just anytime. That doesn't tell you what you want to know. You check your urine first thing in the morning after your body has done its major clean-up from the day before. These results tell you if you have enough neutralizing minerals to keep your internal acid level under control. We'll go into the details of how to carry out and interpret your detective work in Chapter 8.

The urine pH test requires planning. You need to prepare for it by eating particular foods before you do the test. You also need to be clear-headed enough in the morning when you get up to remember to check "the trash" first thing. Since the urine test requires advanced preparation, here are three "tests" that are less precise but sure signs of acid toxicity.

Fist Test

First thing in the morning when you wake up, make a fist. Squeeze. Do you get a lackluster response? Do you feel as though perhaps the "squeeze" message didn't quite make it from your brain to your hand? Is there so little power in your clenched fist that it would leave no blemish on a brand new toothpaste tube? Does squeezing hurt? If all, or any, of the above apply to your fist test, your body is probably more acid than it should be. It's acidotic — toxic.

WELLNESS PRINCIPLE: **A weak or painful fist means too much internal acid.**

Sniff Test

Body waste is made up of the remnants of the foods you have eaten recently and remnants of physiological functions. The waste your body eliminates is a good indicator of how things are going inside. If your stool has a strong odor, or if your urine is "foamy," you've eaten too much protein in the past few days. If your urine smells like ammonia, you've been eating too much protein for too long. A powerful back-up survival system has kicked in. We'll go into the relevance of ammonia at much greater length later on. For the purposes of the "Sniff" test, urine that has an ammonia odor indicates that your body is using a very effective backup system to neutralize dietary acid.

WELLNESS PRINCIPLE: **The odor of ammonia in the urine is a warning sign on the road to disease.**

Stiff Test

Do you start the day feeling "stiff" but "loosen up" as the day goes on? A "Yes" answer means you've been eating too much protein for too long. Your internal environment is fighting protein pollution.

One of the cultural norms of our society is to accept "morning stiffness" as a standard symptom of aging. Early morning creaks and stiffness are passed off as part of the "Ohhhh, I'm getting older" syndrome. They are lumped in with other accepted signs of aging such as waning energy and thinning hair.

Heredity probably has more to do with thinning hair than does diet. But diet has more to do with waning energy and morning stiffness than does heredity. Your morning may begin with your fingers stiff and fumbling as you try to tie your shoes or button your shirt. But they loosen up as the day goes on. That's no big deal, we rationalize. Just getting older.

Well, indeed, you are getting older. But getting older isn't an excuse for every ache and pain. Stiff-in-the-morning-and-better-later is a clue that your body is working overtime to keep your acid levels under control. We can't stop the aging process and continue to live. But we don't have to accelerate the process by dumping a continuous supply of high-protein acid ash-producing foods into our bodies.

WELLNESS PRINCIPLE: Aging is no excuse for stiffness.

If you flunked any or all of the Fist, Sniff, or Stiff tests, your body is toxic from *too much* acid. The "too much" part is from excess dietary protein. There's no instant cure for toxicity. It takes time, commitment, and some new choices on your part. But you can begin today to give your body a break from the acid cycle. Add one serving of *cooked* vegetables to your daily fare. Even if you usually eat no vegetables at all, add only one serving. Not two, or three, or four. Just one serving. Diet changes should be made gradually, especially if your body is extremely toxic. You'll see why, later.

WELLNESS PRINCIPLE: **Quick changes are great for stage shows, but not for diets.**

Your body needs dietary protein to survive. You need enough protein. You don't need too much. Excess protein is the problem, not protein itself. That's a big switch from the usual thinking that more protein is better. More protein means more acid for your body to contend with. Too much protein means too much acid for anyone, and too much protein means way too much acid for those with a waning alkaline reserve.

If you're serious about giving your body the best chance for the best future possible, you won't overburden it with too much protein. Only you can make food choices that will lead to a healthful future. Your body merely works with what you give it. And it doesn't care a bit about the future. It deals only with "the now." Your body doesn't think. It responds. It responds by adjusting the way it's functioning to have the best crack at survival of the moment. Your body doesn't care if you hurt, or have migraines, or have been given three months to live. It doesn't even care if you eat only acid ash-producing foods. It just responds to current conditions, whatever they are. And as current conditions change from what you consider health to what you consider disease, your body responds to those conditions, too. It doesn't plan ahead; you do.

WELLNESS PRINCIPLE: **For your body, the future is now.**

Let's put this acid-alkaline business in whole-body perspective. And in the process, we'll see why your body is *alkaline by design and acid by function*.

CHAPTER 3

COPING WITH THE ACID GENERATION

ALKALINE BY DESIGN

There's just no getting around it. Reading about acid in your body probably isn't the most stimulating, fun-filled, activity. Watching TV cowboys and Indians mix it up on the football field or make-believe battlegrounds, visiting the Grand Canyon, jogging or strolling through nature's wonderlands, weeding your garden, raiding the refrigerator, or pondering the meaning of life are probably much more enjoyable. However, those fun things affect your body for only a short time. What you're reading about could affect your whole life. So it's time to talk a little more about this acid and alkaline business. To get an idea of how acid and alkaline relate to foods you eat, we need to know more than vinegar is acid and baking soda is alkaline.

But take heart; we'll just nibble around the edges of "scientific stuff." Just enough nibbling to introduce you to some internal systems you may not have met before. You may even get a clue as to why you or your family members have persistent, unexplained aches and pains.

Recall that tricky little phrase "*alkaline by design, acid by function*" we have used a couple of times. That's the key! Your cells work best in a slightly alkaline environment, but these same cells produce acid when they work. So your body is constantly making and eliminating acid. It was designed that way.

And the "*alkaline by design, acid by function*" concept is also the key that unlocks the great mystery of why people who eat lots of veggies generally seem to be healthier than those who don't. The reason is that their bodies aren't in damage-control mode trying to subdue excess dietary acid. You see, most vegetables and fruits don't leave hard-to-eliminate acid. On the contrary, most fruits and vegetables leave ingredients that help the body neutralize hard-to-eliminate acid. More veggies and fruit, more acid-fighting nutrients.

WELLNESS PRINCIPLE: Fight acid fallout — eat lots of veggies.

Dietary vegetables help keep your body alkaline. Your cells work best in an internal environment that is slightly alkaline. But we've said that working cells produce acid. Just about everything you do causes your cells to generate internal acid. Eating, breathing, playing golf, scratching your elbow, flicking the TV remote, sumo wrestling. Even thinking! So your body produces acid all the time. It's a standard body response.

Hold it! I can see the question marks glistening in your eyes.

"What about the old 'every response of the body is perfect' concept of a few pages back?" you ask. "If the body responds by producing acid all the time, and every response of the body is perfect, then producing acid must be perfect," you reason.

Good thinking!

Acid production by your body *is* perfect. Self-produced acid is easily eliminated. Acid residue of food is a different story. The acid left by the ash of dietary animal protein is especially bad. And too much "bad" is terrible. There's a big difference between the acid your body produces and the acid leftovers of your lunchtime hamburger. Self-made acid is weak. Hamburger acid is relatively strong. That's the first difference. The second difference is that getting rid of weak self-made acid is a breeze. You get rid of it when you breathe. It's quick and easy. Part of what you exhale is the remnants of the acid your body generates.

WELLNESS PRINCIPLE: **Self-made acid is no big deal — just blow it off.**

Hamburger (and other animal protein) acid is too strong to go out through your lungs. Strong acid travels through your digestive tract to get out of your body. Much of it is processed through the kidneys and is eliminated in your urine. That's why your urine can give you a clue to the acid level of your internal environment. Hence, the urine test we talked about in the previous chapter. More about that later. First, we need to know a little about what we mean by strong acid, weak acid, strong alkali, and weak alkali.

STRENGTH IN NUMBERS

A cidity or alkalinity can be measured. The term "pH" is used to designate the degree of acidity or alkalinity of a substance — water, ammonia, vinegar, battery acid, swimming pool water, blood, whatever. It is pronounced "p" "h" (pea - aech). For some reason (and I suspect it's to give typesetters and proofreaders fits), the term is written with a lower case "p" and upper case "H". It stands for "potential of Hydrogen" and is related to whether Hydrogen ions are gathered in or given off. Now don't let your eyes glaze over here. We'll get only "sciency" enough to help you understand the meaning of the pH numbers we'll use later.

You might think of pH values on a scale similar to a foot-long ruler. But instead of the scale going from 0 at one end to 12 at the other, the pH scale goes from 0 to 14. A substance that registers pH 0 is completely acid. At pH 14, a substance is completely alkaline. Graphically, it looks like this:

Acid						Neutral							Alkaline
0	1	2	3	4	5	6	7	8	9	10	11	12	13	14

Λ

The midpoint of the scale, pH 7.00, indicates "neutral" — neither acid nor alkaline. On the pH scale, numbers lower than 7 indicate acidity. Numbers higher than 7 indicate alkalinity.

The spaces between the whole numbers are divided into tenths, or hundredths — sometimes thousandths if you're being really precise. So you'll find pH values written as tenths, such as 6.5, or

hundredths such as 7.35, or thousandths such as
8.575. Here, we'll deal in tenths or hundredths.

Let's start in the middle at neutral pH 7.00 and go
down. Just to the left of center is pH 6.99 that's just
barely acid. Moving to the left through lower and
lower numbers indicates stronger and stronger acid.
Eventually you get down to super-acid, burn-right-
through-the-container pH 0. Not good stuff to have
around the house. Household bleach is tame by
comparison.

**WELLNESS PRINCIPLE: The lower the pH number, the
stronger the acid.**

Now go the other way. Start at neutral pH 7.00
and go up the scale to the right and you're on the
alkaline side. At pH 7.01 the substance is barely
alkaline. Keep going to higher and higher numbers
and the alkalinity increases. At pH 14 you're up to
super-caustic, burn-right-through the container,
complete alkalinity. Not good stuff to have around the
house. Household ammonia is nowhere near
complete alkalinity, but it's so strong that just the
aroma is potent enough to make you catch your
breath and cough.

**WELLNESS PRINCIPLE: The higher the pH number,
the stronger the alkali.**

No part of your body (or most anything else) can
tolerate any substance that is completely acid or
completely alkaline — or anywhere close to either —
without suffering major damage. Very strong acids
and very strong alkali are very, very harsh.

Your body doesn't do strong acid or strong alkali well. It works best when your internal environment is *just above* pH 7.00 — just to the alkaline side of neutral.

Does that mean that you want the pH of your internal environment to be 8? That's just above 7.

Not necessarily.

The pH scale is finely tuned. Small changes in numbers mean big changes in acidity or alkalinity. The acidity of a substance that starts out at pH 5 becomes ten times more acid if the pH drops to 4. If it continues to drop to pH 3, it's a hundred times (ten times ten) more acid than it was at pH 5. Consequently, a pH change from 5 to 7 is a major leap. You'll see later why this is significant when we talk about the variations in the pH of particular body fluids.

To give you an idea of how small differences in pH numbers make big differences in conditions, your blood pH should normally be between 7.35 and 7.45 — that's a very narrow range in slight alkalinity.

Blood is pH 7.35 when it carries carbon dioxide (an acid) on its way to be eliminated through your lungs. Blood is pH 7.45 after it has been "cleaned up" — it's rid itself of the carbon dioxide and takes on oxygen to deliver to your heart and the rest of your body. As far as survival is concerned, that narrow blood pH range is not negotiable. If your blood pH falls to 6.8, or if it rises to about 8.0, you're on the way out. Your long-term survival is cut to a few hours if your blood pH moves more than about 0.5 to either side of life-sustaining pH 7.35 - 7.45.

WELLNESS PRINCIPLE: **Tiny changes in pH numbers
can mean big changes in
your body.**

Enough of this "pH 101" course. Let's apply it to
what's going on in your body.

FIGHTING OFF AN ACID ATTACK

In previous chapters, we developed a nodding
acquaintance with neutralizing minerals and your
alkaline reserve. These are the minerals that weaken
strong acid left from high-protein foods. So far, we
have introduced several themes:

- Your body is designed to survive.
- Everything your body does is perfect.
- You are *alkaline by design and acid by function*.
- The ideal pH for your internal environment is
  around 7.0.
- Every activity of your body produces acid
  (physiological acid).
- Physiological acid is weak acid that can be
  eliminated through the lungs.
- Dietary animal protein leaves strong acid in
  your body.
- Strong acid from foods must be eliminated
  through the kidneys.
- Strong acid must be neutralized before being
  eliminated from the body.

Okay, the next question, then, is: "How is strong
acid neutralized so it can be eliminated?"

And the answer is: By adding alkalizing elements
that offset the acidity.

Delicate kidney tissue can be burned by strong acid in urine as it makes its way out of the body. So strong acid must be weakened — "neutralized," "alkalized," "buffered." This is one of the body's survival tactics. It's part of your built-in "save the kidneys" program. If you damage your kidneys, your body can't get rid of toxic materials fast enough for the body to survive. That's the purpose of "kidney dialysis" for people whose kidneys have ceased to function effectively — to clean up internal waste products. Without this clean-up capability, the body becomes overwhelmed with acid — a condition known as *acidosis.*

Your body comes equipped with fantastically intricate systems to keep your internal acid level under control. They are called *buffer systems.* You are probably familiar with the assortment of "buffering agents" advertised on TV that are supposed to "relieve acid indigestion." Those products are directed toward neutralizing stomach acid. Your built-in buffer systems, on the other hand, relieve acid "congestion" rather than "indigestion." They keep your innards — delicate organs, tissues, and cells — from being marinated in an internal flood of acid. That's their job. Your buffer systems work together to keep the pH of their common home — your body — within survival limits.

WELLNESS PRINCIPLE: **The job of your systems, organs, cells, and internal processes is to survive.**

In the survival game, your body's first line of defense against unwelcome or unnecessary intruders is dilution. Water it down and send it out of the body.

We've already seen that weak acid is eliminated through the lungs. Weak acid from alkaline ash vegetables and fruits, from exercise, and from cellular activity is converted to carbon dioxide and out it goes with every moist breath.

When dilution can't do the trick — as with strong acid, your buffer systems get into the act. For our purposes, we'll deal principally with the Big Three buffer systems: the *bicarbonate buffer system*, the *phosphate buffer system*, and the *protein buffer system*. Now you'll see why we went through all of that pH folderol.

Keep in mind that the objective of buffering is to keep your cells happy and productive by keeping the acid in your internal environment under control. And what's the *ideal* pH of your internal environment? You've got it — *about* pH 7.0. Here's a condensed version (not a textbook version) of how your buffer systems work to reduce "acid pollution" in and around your cells.

Bicarbonate Buffer System

The bicarbonate buffer system works outside the cells — extracellularly. Its principal acid-fighters are sodium and bicarbonate. The bicarb system is the part of your acid defense team that jumps into action first. It's the "first responder." It can get things started, but it can't do the whole job. The bicarbonate buffer system isn't as powerful as the phosphate and protein systems. The bicarb system can't raise internal pH as close to alkalinity as the phosphate and protein systems can. The bicarb system handles the first wave of an acid attack launched by dietary animal protein.

To illustrate how your survival-oriented body marshals its buffer systems to protect you from the consequences of inappropriate food choices, we'll use the example of your lunchtime hamburger. Here's the scene your bicarbonate buffer system faces.

You have just eaten lunch: A juicy quarter-pounder, a dab of condiments, a bit of lettuce, a slice of tomato, pickle, and onion, nestled in a bun. This jaw-stretching treat is ordinarily accompanied by the traditional fries and diet carbonated soft drink (pop or soda, depending on the part of the country you're from). As lunches go, it was fast, convenient, and tasted pretty good even though the Heart Association might call it "the heart attack special."

Okay, now you've eaten it; your body must do something with it — use it or lose it.

Remember that, in general, meat, fish, poultry, and grains are acid ash producers, and vegetables and fruits are alkaline ash producers. From the acid perspective, there's not enough lettuce, tomato, and pickle accompanying your lunchtime hamburger to affect the acid-alkaline picture one way or another. The fries are on the "plus" side. They are alkaline ash-producers. The bun and the condiments could be slightly on the negative side. However, the meat patty — all four ounces of it — is high-protein stuff. It leaves a lot of strong acid that can burn delicate tissues and membranes and send your extracellular pH plummeting to crisis level. So what happens?

Bicarbonate buffer system to the rescue! It may not be powerful, but it's effective. In a flash, the bicarb system deploys its alkaline reserve forces — bicarbonate and sodium — to go to work on the attacking acid. Sodium is a key player. So when the bicarb and sodium jump in to the acid environment,

their alkalinity begins to neutralize the strong acid —
the pH edges up closer to neutral.

With the strong acid forces of your hamburger's
acid ash subdued by your sodium defenders, the
extracellular pH level rises. But your bicarb buffer
system can't do the whole job. It can raise the pH to
only 6.1. However, that's good enough to reduce the
threat to your cells of too much acid in their external
environment. Whew! That was close. Without the aid
of your bicarbonate buffer system forces, your whole
internal environment could have been fatally
polluted.

Unfortunately, repelling this acid attack was not
without casualties. In the process of the fray, some of
your sodium forces sacrificed themselves.

"Sacrificed themselves?"

Right. A little respect, please, for the sodium
elements that helped assure your body's survival for
another nanosecond. They gave up their cozy
existence in your internal environment to escort
dangerous acid out of your body to who-knows-
where. However, this is not exactly an act of courage.
It's a response. Sodium doesn't think. Your body
doesn't think. Your systems don't think. Your cells
don't think. And the elements that make up all of the
above don't think. They respond. And when there's
strong acid "attacking" your internal environment,
the response includes using all the available sodium
necessary to weaken the acid so your body can get
rid of it.

We have said that acid from hamburger (and other
dietary animal protein) is too strong to be eliminated
through the lungs. It must be eliminated through the
kidneys. But it must be toned down first or it will
damage the kidneys on the way through. Once the

sodium and bicarbonate have tamed the hamburger acid, they stay with it all the way out of the body. That means that every time you have a hamburger or other acid ash-producing tasty for lunch, breakfast, dinner or snack, part of your alkaline reserve — principally sodium — is "sacrificed" to buffer the acid. The hero of the day is sodium. Not salt — sodium. So don't pepper your food with salt thinking you're helping it out. You aren't, but right now we're doing buffer systems. We'll talk about the difference between sodium and salt later.

WELLNESS PRINCIPLE: Strong acid in, neutralizing sodium out.

However, that's not the end of the situation. Your sodium sacrifice took care of the immediate problem. It raised your internal environment from "way-too-acid" to a "too-acid" pH 6.1. Your internal Environmental Protection Agency insists that your blood pH stays in the neighborhood of 7.3. It won't stand for an environment as sloppy as pH 6.1. That's not good enough for inside your cells.

Enter the phosphate buffer system.

Phosphate Buffer System

The phosphate buffer system works intracellularly — inside the cells. The principal buffering agent of the phosphate buffer system is potassium. There's more potassium inside the cells than outside. No matter what's going on outside the cells' walls, most of the potassium will stay inside the cells to do its job. And one of its most important jobs is to raise the pH of fluids inside the cell as high as it can, which is pH 6.8.

WELLNESS PRINCIPLE: The phosphate buffer system begins clean-up operations inside the cell.

On with our story.

Outside the cells, the hamburger acid has now been subdued — not conquered, but subdued. The pH of your outside-the-cell environment is still a zippy 6.1. That's not good enough for inside the cells. And the atmosphere outside the cells affects the atmosphere inside the cells. The phosphate buffer system can raise the pH of intracellular fluid from 6.1 to 6.8. But blood needs to be in the pH 7.35 - 7.45 range. So the phosphate buffer system helps combat the acid attack, but can't finish the job. The phosphate system takes the pH only to 6.8. It still needs to get up over pH 7.0. That's the job of the protein buffer system.

The Protein Buffer System

The protein buffer system is the most powerful of the three buffer systems. It handles most of the buffering in the body — about 75%.

If it's so powerful and does most of the buffering, why do we need the bicarbonate and phosphate systems? Seems like there's some duplication of effort here.

And there would be if the buffer systems were generalists instead of specialists. Although the three systems work together, each has a well defined job description. Each works in its own area of expertise. The bicarb buffer, with sodium as its principal acid-fighter, can take strong acid up to pH 6.1. The phosphate buffer, with potassium leading the charge, can take the pH 6.1 acid up to pH 6.8. The protein buffer is an expert at taking the pH from 6.8 to 7.4. That's our goal. But hamburger acid is too strong for the protein system to handle from start to finish.

WELLNESS PRINCIPLE: The protein buffering system fine-tunes pH.

Like the phosphate system, the protein buffer system operates inside the cell. However, the protein system doesn't need a "partner," such as sodium or potassium, the way the bicarbonate and phosphate systems do. The protein does it all itself.

Ooops! Have we just come up with a contradiction? We've been saying that protein causes acid. Now we're saying that protein buffers acid. What's the deal?

Two things.

First, the limited range of the protein buffer. It can't do its job unless the acid is very weak — pH 6.8. It can't handle strong hamburger acid straight out of the patty.

Second, protein can work both sides of the street. We said earlier that pH is the potential of Hydrogen — the ability of a substance to gather in, or get rid of, Hydrogen ions. Well, protein is a living structure that can do both. It can change the position of its atoms and either attract or repel Hydrogen ions. So it can both acidify and neutralize.

But if there's too much protein in the cells, there's more acid in the cells than the protein buffers can handle. Too many hamburgers in your diet will eventually mean too much acid in your cells, and too much acid in your cells means you've been making some wrong choices.

When we talk about the perils of dietary protein, we're talking about too much protein. Excess dietary protein. The worst offender is dietary animal protein. But, as we'll see, eating too much of any kind of protein is body abuse. *Too much* dietary protein creates more acid ash than the three buffers combined can handle.

WELLNESS PRINCIPLE: We need protein — we don't need *too much* protein.

So we've come full circle. Your digested lunchtime hamburger set into motion the buffering action of all three buffering systems. They work together to keep both the internal environment where your cells live — and your cells themselves — at the best pH possible.

All right. That's all very interesting and informative. Now, what does it have to do with the grand scheme of things?

That depends on just which "grand scheme" you're talking about. If it's the movement of the constellations or whether or not the U.S. should send troops to the latest global hot spot, the answer is "Not much." But if you're talking about the grand scheme of your life and health, it could mean a difference in your future — a big difference.

The whole diet issue hinges on your alkaline reserve's supply of good usable sodium. Not just how much fat you eat. Not just cholesterol. Not just calories. Sodium! And your supply of good usable sodium depends on how much acid ash-producing food you eat, and how long you've been eating that much.

Acid ash-producing foods aren't all bad. Your body is designed to take care of the acid from foods. It's *too much* high-protein for *too long* that is a problem.

Eating too much protein won't kill you — quickly. But it keeps your body in high gear constantly. That's exhausting. It's exhausting not only for you as a whole, but for your component parts — the organs, systems, and cells that keep you going. No organ or system can function at top speed constantly without breaking down. So, after a while, something "breaks down." Then you have a name to hang onto the "broken down" area: heart attack, arthritis, osteoporosis, chronic fatigue syndrome, diabetes, or whatever. However, the symptoms are so far removed from your breakfast eggs, lunchtime hamburgers, and dinner lamb pilaf that it's difficult to make the connection. But the connection is there.

WELLNESS PRINCIPLE: **Disease follows exhaustion, and exhaustion follows coping with too much dietary protein.**

There's not much point in talking about "too much" protein if we don't know how much is enough. So, let's find out how much we need and how much is too much.

SOME COMMON ALKALINE ASH FOODS
(Help to control acid in your internal environment)

Almonds	Dates, dried	Parsnips
Apples	Figs, dried	Peaches
Apricots	Grapefruit	Pears
Avocados	Grapes	Pineapple
Bananas	Green beans	Potatoes, sweet
Beans, dried	Green peas	Potatoes, white
Beet greens	Lemons	Radishes
Beets	Lettuce	Raisins
Blackberries	Lima beans, dried	Raspberries
Broccoli	Lima beans, green	Rhubarb**
Brussels sprouts	Limes	Rutabagas
Cabbage	Milk, goat*	Sauerkraut
Carrots	Millet	Soy beans, green
Cauliflower	Molasses	Spinach, raw
Celery	Mushrooms	Strawberries
Chard leaves	Muskmelons	Tangerines
Cherries, sour	Onions	Tomatoes
Cucumbers	Oranges	Watercress
		Watermelon

*   Recommended for infants only when mother's milk
    is not available
** Not recommended: has properties detrimental to the
    body

SOME COMMON ACID ASH FOODS
(Leave strong acid in your internal environment)

Bacon	Eggs	Pork
Barley grain	Flour, white	Prunes^
Beef	Flour, whole wheat	Rice, brown
Blueberries	Haddock	Rice, white
Bran, wheat	Honey	Salmon
Bran, oat	Lamb	Sardines
Bread, white	Lentils, dried	Sausage
Bread, whole wheat	Lobster	Scallops
Butter	Milk, cow's^	Shrimp
Carob	Macaroni	Spaghetti
Cheese	Oatmeal	Squash, winter
Chicken	Oysters	Sunflower seeds
Cod	Peanut butter	Turkey
Corn	Peanuts	Veal
Corned beef	Peas, dried	Walnuts
Crackers, soda	Pike	Wheat germ
Cranberries	Plums^	Yogurt
Currants		

^ These foods leave an alkaline ash but have an acidifying effect on the body.

NEUTRAL ASH FOODS THAT HAVE
AN ACIDIFYING EFFECT

Corn oil	Corn syrup	Olive oil	Refined sugar

CHAPTER 4

ACID ON THE HOOF

HOW MUCH IS TOO MUCH?

There's no point in talking about "too much protein" if we don't know how much is enough. Most of us grew up accepting the adage: "You can't get too much protein." Super-high protein weight-loss programs were the "in thing" several years ago. But people died from these. So these programs fell out of favor. Folks get testy when their loved ones die from using a product that was supposed to help them lose weight and increase energy.

Protein has an energizing effect. Protein is stimulating. It revs up your body and you enjoy the benefits of the increased energy. But it's a temporary rev as your body shifts into overdrive to handle the acid. Acid is a threat to survival. When your body is warding off an "attack," your energy level increases. Yet the aftermath of the survival game is an energy-drain. So, you need to eat more protein to get going again. With the "more protein," you get more acid.

And the cycle repeats itself. In the process, your
alkaline reserve takes a beating.

The human body is by far the most sophisticated
piece of "machinery" ever devised. Compared to the
body, the most advanced computers are Tinker Toys.
Our bodies' survival mechanisms are designed and
constructed in such a way that they can overcome
just about any fool thing we do to them — at least for
a while. One of the biggest "fool things" we do to our
bodies is to eat too much of the food that keeps our
survival systems going full tilt constantly — high-
protein meat, poultry, fish, and grains.

We know that protein is the foundation of the
building blocks of the cells. Proteins in the body are
constantly "lost" as they are "degraded" to be used
again by the body. Every day, we use and replace
about 20 to 30 grams of protein. Much of the
replacement protein comes from food. So, how much
protein do you need to eat to replace the losses and
keep your body in good working order? How much is
too much?

Recommendations for "ideal" quantities of
dietary protein, carbohydrates (sugar and starch
producers), or fat are generally given in grams —
usually written gm, or g. A gram isn't a whole lot. It's
equal to about three-hundredths (more precisely,
0.03215) of an ounce. You can mail 28 of these little
rascals with one first-class stamp. Minerals, on the
other hand, are referred to in smaller quantities.
Mineral recommendations are usually given in
milligrams — mg — one-thousandth of a gram. It
takes a thousand milligrams to make one gram. We're
talking small quantities here. Back to the "how
much."

The amount of daily protein recommended as "should have" has changed over the years. Around the end of the 19th century, the recommendation was 118 gm of protein a day. The story behind how researchers settled on this number is that they measured the amount of protein consumed daily by a group of healthy young men. Apparently the reasoning was that if these young men were healthy, they were eating the right amount of protein. But time and science march on.

By 1965, either our needs or our knowledge changed. The recommended amount dropped from 118 gm to 70 gm for men and 58 gm for women in the 35 - 75 year age group. But it didn't stop there. In the 1970s and '80s, not only the amount recommended by the US government changed but the age groupings also changed. The recommendation for males 15 - 51+ years old was 56 gm; for 19 - 51+ year-old females it was 44 gm.

WELLNESS PRINCIPLE: **Daily protein requirements weren't specified on the tablets that came down from the mountain.**

As you can see, the recommended amount keeps dropping. Today, some authorities suggest that our daily protein intake should be limited to 20 gm. This is probably close to ideal. However, as a practical matter, you can "get by" with up to 40 gm a day as long as all of those protein grams march hand-in-hand through your digestive system with neutralizing fruits and vegetables.

Let's take a look at how your now famous lunchtime hamburger stacked up according to protein requirements.

	Grams of Protein
3 oz. hamburger patty -	
broiled - 3" x 5/8" - lean	21
hamburger roll	3
tomato slice	trace
lettuce	trace
Total	24+ a couple of traces

You've already topped 24 gm and you haven't even started on your french fries. Ten french fries, 2 - 3 1/2 inches long, fried in vegetable oil, add another 2 gm. Now you're just over 26 gm. You could have lowered that by one gram if you'd gone for a regular fat-dripping hamburger instead of a "low fat" lean hamburger. But if you splurge and have a slice of cheese on your burger, you get another 6 gm. That's 32 gm of protein for lunch. What about breakfast? If you had an egg cooked in butter (6 gm) and a piece of whole wheat toast (3 gm), you've topped 40 gm of protein. And dinner's yet to come.

LEAN, MEAN PROTEIN

In our society today, we focus more on dietary fat and cholesterol than on protein. Thousands of people methodically count fat grams each day and meal. That's the "in" thing. Fat is the big, fat, bugaboo of health, we're told. Cut down on the amount of fat you get, we hear and read, and you'll

cut down your chances of developing heart disease
and other modern-day life-threateners. And they are
right. But for the wrong reason.

This is another example of mistaking symptoms
for cause. Sure, dietary fat is a major factor in artery-
clogging heart disease. And that can kill you. But the
fat's not the grass-roots problem. The cause of the
problem is what carries the fat. High-protein flesh
foods. Meat, poultry, fish, dairy products, and the
many derivatives thereof. In order to lower fat intake,
we lower our animal protein intake. The results may
or may not be the same.

WELLNESS PRINCIPLE: **Less dietary protein, less
                                acid, less internal
                                pollution, less disease.**

One method of cutting down on dietary fat is to
eat lean meat. We are encouraged to buy lean cuts of
meat and to cut the fat off the chubby cuts before
cooking. You can see what this means when you look
at meat and poultry from an acid perspective. Instead
of buying a pound of fat-drenched hamburger, you
buy a pound of lean protein-drenched hamburger.
The same amount of burger; more protein. That's why
when we calculated the protein content of your
lunchtime hamburger we could subtract a gram of
protein if we substituted a regular, fat-filled burger
for the lean. However, this fatty hamburger vs. lean
hamburger comparison is just an illustration. I am
certainly not recommending that you eat fatty meats!

We're not accustomed to holding our protein
intake to under 40 gm. It can be done, but not by
having hamburgers for lunch every day — unless
that's the only meal you have. That's not such a red

hot idea either. To help you keep your protein intake under control, some suggested menus are offered later in this book. When you keep your protein intake under control, you have taken one giant step in keeping dietary stress on your body under control.

Keep in mind that the purpose of holding down protein consumption is to help keep your internal environment a neat place for your cells to live and work. And the effect of a neat internal environment is that it keeps your body from inching slowly but surely into acidosis — which is shorthand for saying "inching slowly but surely into exhaustion, discomfort, pain, and disease."

WELLNESS PRINCIPLE: **"Happy" cells are healthy cells.**

Very likely, we don't *need* any more than 20 gm of protein a day. Your body can tolerate up to 40 grams — as long as you include enough fruits and vegetables in your daily diet to help your body handle the acid residue. However, I'm not convinced that we were created to be gram counters. It doesn't seem logical that our health-determining acid level would hinge on us performing precise mathematical calculations at each meal. A more logical approach is to make sure that at least 70 to 75 percent of everything you eat each day is alkaline ash-producing foods. To put it another way, at meals, three-quarters of the food on your meal plates should be alkaline ash-producing. That leaves you up to 25 to 30 percent to do with as you please. The lists of common alkaline ash and acid ash foods on pages 51 and 52 should help you.

WELLNESS PRINCIPLE: **Eat hearty while you eat healthy.**

When you follow the 70% - 30% rule, you can include some acid-ash producing favorites without garnishing them with a ladle full of guilt.

Since you have probably been oblivious to the need for shielding your body from too many acid-producing foods, laying a guilt-trip on yourself for past protein indiscretions is pointless. Most of us do the best we can with the information at hand. Now that you have been exposed to the concept that you can get too much protein, it's still pointless to do the guilt thing if you occasionally err and stray over the acceptable protein limit. Guilt is as hard on your body as excess protein. But, that's another book.

OVER THE LIMIT

Let's look at some of the repercussions of exceeding your protein limit.

We've seen that too much dietary protein litters your innards with strong acid that must be neutralized. And we know that sodium is the mineral of choice for the bicarbonate buffer system's neutralizing job. Sodium comes as part of our standard equipment package. But it's rather like the first tank of gas supplied with a new car. Once used, it must be replaced. The farther you drive (the older you get), the more gas you've used. The more protein you eat, the more sodium you use. Too bad you don't have a "sodium gauge" that's as easy to read as a gas gauge to let you know you've gone too far without "refueling."

Sodium is one of the most important elements in your body. It does some wonderful things, and you never know they are happening. Sodium is the principal positively charged element in extracellular fluid. Sodium salts (as they are called) are important ingredients in serum, blood, and lymph. They also maintain a balance between calcium and potassium to maintain normal heart action and the pressure in cells and fluids. And to top it off, sodium salts guard against excessive loss of water from tissues.

WELLNESS PRINCIPLE: **Sodium is one essential dude.**

All of the many jobs sodium quietly performs in your body are geared toward immediate survival. Only sodium can perform some of these functions. How's that for job security?

So what happens when sodium is constantly called on to "sacrifice itself" by neutralizing an unrelenting acid attack of excess protein? After a while, the sodium contingent dwindles and there aren't enough sodium replacements. Sure enough, there's still sodium in the body. But those sodium troops are wrapped up in other high-priority missions, like keeping the heart beating properly and maintaining proper pressure of extracellular fluid and cells.

Back to your bicarbonate buffer system to pull this all together. Your bicarb system is your first line of defense against strong dietary acid. Every time you eat animal protein, your body calls on the sodium and bicarbonate of your alkaline reserve. This isn't a big problem as far as the bicarb is concerned; your body keeps that in constant supply. However, your usable sodium supply is another story. Your body doesn't make sodium. It gathers it along with other minerals from incoming fruits and vegetables. Unfortunately, for all too many people in our country, their bodies have barely a nodding acquaintance with carrots, apples, green beans, oranges, broccoli, or other "live foods" that offer suitable sodium replacements. After a while the sodium in their alkaline reserve begins to dwindle. With sodium forces dwindling, the bicarb system's initial strike force in the war against strong acid is seriously "under-mineraled." Strong acid continues to attack. Excess acid is still a serious threat to the body. What's a body to do?

The body does just what any good commander would do: call up able-bodied replacements from jobs less survival specific. Bicarb can't buffer by itself. The body's in a pinch. It can't live with the acid, but it can live without attending to tasks that aren't essential to immediate survival — rebuilding bones, healing wounds, keeping gallbladder bile liquid enough so stones don't form, and other nice but non-survival processes. Sodium and other neutralizing minerals that are performing these routine maintenance jobs are called on to replace the dwindling forces of the alkaline reserve. Routine maintenance can wait. Acid will be neutralized!

The replacement mineral most called on is calcium. And where is most of the calcium stored in your body? Right! Teeth and bones.

When your acid-neutralizing sodium supply has dwindled to crisis level, the calcium stored in your bones is the next-best neutralizer. You can live quite a while without strong bones. Bones that become fragile enough to snap, crackle, and pop may be inconvenient and painful. But inconvenient and painful aren't fatal. They are merely irksome and hurtsome. Brittle or porous bones are an effect of your problem, not the problem itself. They are an effect of your body responding perfectly to survive a continuous torrent of strong, life-threatening dietary acid.

> **WELLNESS PRINCIPLE:**   **Puny bones beat death by acid.**

The solution to this problem seems obvious: If a shortage of sodium and calcium are behind major physical problems, eat more salt and drink more milk.

That would be great, if it worked. However, as Gilbert and Sullivan put it, "Things are seldom as they seem. . . ."

THE GREAT IMPERSONATOR

The sodium your body uses isn't the same as the salt you put on your eggs or french fries. That's sodium chloride. You get sodium chloride out of a salt shaker, on pretzels and potato chips, in fast foods, and in canned soups and other processed foods. Sodium chloride adds zest to the taste of foods. If food comes from a can, a box, or a restaurant, chances are excellent that it comes with a lot of sodium your body can't use. As you will see in the next chapter, the sodium your body uses has been processed through plants — it's organic sodium.

Your body uses organic minerals that come apart easily. Table salt isn't organic sodium. Table salt hasn't been processed through living plants. It comes from the ground. It's about 40% sodium and 60% chloride. The sodium and chloride that make up table salt are held together tightly. The bond is rather like that of chewing gum in a kid's hair — two separate and distinct entities locked firmly together. The sodium and chloride are so tightly connected that the sodium can't be easily released to join the buffering crowd. It can't join the ranks of the other internal sodium workers. However, sodium chloride resembles its organic sodium cousin so closely that the body can be fooled into letting it stay. Remember the "use it or lose it" motto of the body? Salt can get around that by impersonating the good stuff. Consequently, the body doesn't send it packing.

Although it can't be used as a buffering agent, sodium chloride can stay in the blood stream and affect the "pressure" balance of cells. This is the sodium that heart patients are advised to restrict. The sodium in fruits and vegetables is good stuff.

WELLNESS PRINCIPLE: **Table salt doesn't fortify your alkaline reserve.**

Table salt is a preservative and a condiment. It serves very useful purposes. A little salt enhances the flavor of foods. But, like protein, you don't need a lot of it. Evidence is beginning to surface that for every teaspoon of salt consumed (about 2,000 mg of sodium) significant amounts of calcium are lost in urine. Calcium loss can be a particular problem if calcium is already being siphoned from your bones to help neutralize high-protein acid.

Okay, if there's not enough calcium, milk is the answer. Right? Not quite . . . .

OSTEOPOROSIS BY THE QUART

J ust as the sodium in table salt isn't a substitute for organic sodium, the calcium in pasteurized cow's milk isn't a substitute for organic calcium. Drinking more milk won't increase a waning calcium supply. In fact, drinking more milk compounds the problem.

We have been led to believe that if we drink a glass of milk every day we can ward off the threat of creeping osteoporosis. However, that doesn't track with studies that correlate calcium consumption with hip fractures.

Hip fractures can be an indicator of brittle bones.

A study published in 1986 showed the incidence of hip fractures in relation to the consumption of calcium and protein. The author of the article observed that a positive relationship exists between protein intake and hip fractures, and that in populations where calcium intake is relatively high and dairy products are common, hip fractures are more common. The author of the article says, ". . . there are *no* [his emphasis] data available to demonstrate that high calcium intakes do, in fact, help prevent osteoporosis." And more startling, the author points out "that hip fractures and protein intake are positively related, and obviously there is a positive correlation between calcium and protein consumption."[1]

Results from ten countries were included in the study. The results were impressive. If the researchers had awarded medals to the countries with the highest incidence of hip fractures, the United States would have won the gold in both the calcium and protein consumption divisions. The United States tallied about 100 hip fractures per 100,000 people. In contrast, Singapore and Hong Kong had the lowest number of hip fractures at about 30 per 100,000 people. But they are at a definite disadvantage in the great hip fracture break-off: they consume considerably less calcium and protein than we do.

Other research also links protein with calcium loss (then we'll leave the studies to the textbooks). A 1973 study was conducted with "nine young adult human males" — that means college students. These young males consumed 500 mg of calcium daily (that's less than the recommended amount of 800 mg). At different points in the study, the young men consumed different amounts of protein: 47 gm, 95 gm, and 142 gm of protein daily. (Keep in mind here that the government recommends 56 gm of protein a day for men.) At the low of 47 gm of protein, two of the nine lost more calcium in their urine and feces than they consumed. When the subjects consumed 95 gm or more of protein and increased their fruit and vegetable intake by 50% they lost more calcium than they consumed. The more protein they ate, the more calcium they lost. When they had more than 47 gm of protein a day, it didn't make any difference how much vegetables and fruits they ate. They still lost more calcium than they took in.

WELLNESS PRINCIPLE: **Eat great gobs of protein and even fruits and vegetables can't come to your rescue.**

What does that have to do with milk?

You'll notice that milk shows up on the list of acid ash foods. Cow's milk leaves an alkaline ash, but it has an acidifying effect on your body.

Huh? Alkaline ash, acidifying effect? That doesn't seem right.

But it is. The explanation revolves around phosphorus and the amount of protein. Milk contains phosphorus. We need phosphorus. Phosphorus compounds are a principal source of energy in muscle contraction and in converting food to energy. But phosphorus is acidifying.

Here's an interesting situation. Mother's milk — nature's truly perfect food, for babies — also contains phosphorus. Yet mother's milk doesn't acidify a baby's body. The difference between cow's milk and mother's milk is the ratio of calcium to phosphorus. Mother's milk has over twice as much calcium as phosphorus — it has 2 calciums to 1 phosphorus. Cow's milk has only about one and a quarter times as much calcium as phosphorus — 1.25 calcium to 1 phosphorus. And then there's the protein factor again. Human milk contains 1.1 mg of protein compared with 3.5 mg of protein in the same amount of cow's milk. Just handling the protein in cow's milk generates acid in the body.

The upshot of all of this is that the more milk you drink, the more protein and acid your body must contend with, the more calcium you lose, and the more likely you are to develop osteoporosis or some other degenerative disease. So, if you are intent on keeping your bones as strong and sturdy as possible, and you are intent on living as pain-free a life as possible, you'll keep your protein intake around 40 gm or less a day and avoid drinking milk. If your internal workings could think and speak, they'd thank you for it.

Increasing numbers of "experts" are coming to understand the concept I have been preaching for over twenty years: most of our physical ills aren't products of consuming too little body-building protein, they are products of consuming too much. That's why the "experts" advise you to eat more fruits and vegetables. Many of them may still not understand "why," they just know it works. So, let's look at what lowly plant foods have to offer.

CHAPTER 5

VIM, VIGOR, AND VEGGIES

ACID DAMAGE CONTROL

Now that the character of hamburger, milk, and other dietary animal protein has been assailed, let's look at the role of fruits and vegetables in our day-to-day lives and health.

With all of our wonderful buffer systems at work for us day and night, one might think that our cells would languish contentedly in a sublimely acid-free body. If that were the case, we would all be robust, energetic, pain-free, and peace would reign throughout the world. Well, maybe not the peace part, but at least we'd feel better and we'd have more energy.

We know that when we eat animal protein, our sophisticated buffer systems pitch right in to weaken strong acid. And we know that, in the process, valuable minerals — sodium, calcium, and whatever else is needed for acid damage control — are lost. So it stands to reason that we should replace those minerals at every opportunity. And the biggest opportunities are meal times.

You make essential health-determining choices every day. Your body must survive the effects of these choices. So you may as well make food choices that help your body survive without working itself to death. Fruits and vegetables are the foods of choice in this category. They are, in general, alkaline ash-producing foods. Alkaline ash includes minerals that help keep the acid level of your body under control. That's what overall health is all about — getting and keeping your internal environment at a comfortable slightly alkaline pH. The most appropriate food choices are those that allow your body to enjoy a slightly alkaline internal environment.

WELLNESS PRINCIPLE: **Vegetables and fruits are easy-response, minimum-stress foods.**

Vegetables and fruits are easily digested. They contribute more to the body than they use. Most of them don't reduce your alkaline reserve — they are major contributors to your acid-neutralizing brigade. And they don't have cholesterol or a lot of fat in them — a real plus for fat-gram and cholesterol counters.

Fruits and vegetables provide a host of internal workers — vitamins, minerals, amino acids, and cellulose. Vitamins, minerals, and amino acids help nourish your cells. They are tools your body needs to repair and replenish itself. Cellulose is a different story.

Cellulose is plant fiber — the stuff that supports the framework of the plant. Your body can't use cellulose. It can't change the components of cellulose into usable nutrients. Well, then, if the body can't use it, we don't need it, do we?

Actually, cellulose has a very important job in your body. The job of cellulose is to provide bulk to shepherd waste materials, such as food residue, spent cells and bacteria, out of the body. That's one of the major advantages touted by the "eat more veggies but I'm not sure why" clan — to keep the elimination process active and to avoid, or overcome, constipation. Big cellulose contributors include (but are not limited to) apples, apricots, asparagus, beans, beets, bran flakes, broccoli, cabbage, celery, mushrooms, oatmeal, onions, oranges, parsnips, prunes, spinach, turnips, wheat flakes, whole grains, and whole wheat bread. Hhhmmm. Sounds like the stuff you should be eating anyway. Chalk-up another point for fruits and veggies.

More good news. Fruits and vegetables bring with them their own self-processing enzymes. Enzymes act as catalysts. They make things happen. They are complex proteins, produced by living cells. They can cause chemical changes in other substances without being changed themselves. You produce enzymes and you consume enzymes.

You have bunches of enzymes in your body. Enzymes with strange-sounding names "splash about" in internal fluids — ptyalin in saliva; pepsins, gelatinase and lipase in gastric (stomach) juice; trypsin, chymotrypsin, amylopsin and others in pancreatic juice; erepsin, amylase, enterokinase and company in intestinal juice, and nucleosidases in mucous. Different enzymes have different jobs. Some change starch to sugar. Some help digest food. Some change emulsified fats of cream and egg yolk into fatty acids. Some divide amino acids into ammonia compounds. And some spark chemical changes in the cells.

When you eat a ripe apple or green salad, you get enzymes along with a fresh supply of minerals. Keep in mind, however, that heating destroys enzymes. Enzymes help in digesting the food that brought them. The minerals help to keep your internal environment clean, neat, and unpolluted. It's rather like having enjoyable house guests who scrub the bathrooms, do the laundry, rake the leaves, wash the car, and leave coupons for prepaid Happy Housecleaners services.

WELLNESS PRINCIPLE: **Fruits and vegetables pay their way.**

Most fruit and some vegetables come equipped with more than just vitamins, minerals, and enzymes. Acid. Plucked right off the plant, most fruits are highly acid. Test most fresh fruit with pH paper and it registers acid. Even apparently mild-mannered fresh pears weigh in on the pH scale at below 5.5. Citrus fruits, such as lemons, grapefruit, and oranges are noticeably acid. They contain citric acid. Apples contain malic acid. If we're trying to keep our bodies from being too acid, wouldn't fruit be the first thing to go?

Not necessarily.

Even though the fruit acid is strong, tangy, and tart in your mouth, it acidifies your body only temporarily. Fruit acid is *organic* acid — the kind that is easily broken down and eliminated through the lungs. Whew!

However, some people have problems when they eat any kind of fruit. You're probably beginning to see why. Their bodies are already too acid to comfortably handle an additional sudden acid surge. Although the acid in fruit is easily eliminated through the lungs, it doesn't get the bum's rush. It takes a few minutes for the acid to make its way through the discharge process. In the meantime, the quick rush of fruit acid brings on unpleasant but temporary symptoms. There's nothing wrong with the acid in the fruit. The problem is that the person's acid level is already maxed out. In addition, his or her acid-fighting forces are plumb-tuckered-out from waging a non-stop campaign against excess dietary protein. Those who can't handle the "hard stuff" of naturally acid raw fruit need to begin a deacidifying campaign by adding a serving of mild-mannered cooked vegetables to their daily menu.

Most fruits and some veg are very acid on their way into the body. But they have an alkalizing effect once they get in. If your body is really overly acidic — if you flunked the fist, sniff, or stiff tests — start bringing your pH level up with cooked veg, not raw fruit.

NATURE'S NUTRIENT FACTORIES

Adequate supplies of neutralizing minerals are essential to keep our internal environments in tip-top shape. We get a variety of minerals and other nutrients when we eat a variety of foods. Virtually all foods have minerals and other nutrients — even acid ash foods. The question is: Why are vegetable and fruit minerals better than meat, poultry, fish, and cheese minerals?

The answer is: Plants get minerals straight from the ground. These minerals are processed by the plants. When we eat the plants, the minerals are ready for our bodies to use. Minerals we get from meat, poultry, and other flesh foods are at least one step further removed from their origin. The animal or fish or other move-abouts get minerals from plants they eat. But that doesn't mean the minerals are suitable for our bodies. By the time you eat the meat, the alkalizing plant minerals — sodium, calcium, potassium, magnesium, and iron — have already been processed through another body. In addition, the meat brings along with it whole bunches of acidifying minerals — phosphorus, chlorine, sulfur, nitrogen. The acidifying minerals "outweigh" the neutralizing minerals. And that's from meat straight off the hoof. What about the "further processed" meats and derivatives? Cheese, for example, is a by-product of the animal kingdom. Cheese is one of the finer taste treats in life, but it has been through several processes before you eat it.

Fruits and vegetables, on the other hand, work with the raw materials of minerals from the ground, and we reap the benefit of their labor.

WELLNESS PRINCIPLE: **Fruits are alkalizing cocktails with a twist.**

The molecules of the minerals as they come from the ground are held together too tightly for our bodies to break apart and use. Our bodies can't use most minerals as they come from the soil, but plants can. You might say that fruits and vegetables are "first responders." Plants "eat" the minerals in the soil. In the plant, the minerals are processed, or restructured. Then we — and cows, chickens, pigs, deer, turkeys, and sheep — eat parts of the plants and get the reconstructed minerals. When you eat the cow or other animal that has eaten the plant, you get the neutralizing plant minerals remaining in the tissue of the meat. For example, your lunch hamburger has 9 mg of calcium. That sounds pretty good until you compare it with a carrot that has 19 mg of calcium. And the hamburger also has acidifying elements characteristic of high protein animal tissue, such as 134 mg of acidifying phosphorus. The carrot wins again here. It has only 32 mg of phosphorus.

Plants that live in rich soil take nutrients and minerals from the ground through their roots. Plant menus are made up principally of carbon, hydrogen, oxygen, phosphorus, potassium, nitrogen, calcium, iron, magnesium, and small amounts of other elements. These minerals are essentially inorganic — they occur in nature independent of living things. Inorganic minerals are of little use to your body. Their parts are too tightly connected to be easily separated. It's the old gum-in-kid's-hair syndrome. Your body works best with "gum-free" organic minerals that separate easily.

WELLNESS PRINCIPLE: **Inorganic minerals are broken down in natures' best processing plants.**

In the plant, inorganic elements are incorporated into organic molecules. We might say that the difference between inorganic and organic is like the difference between super glue and Velcro. Super glue holds tightly — Velcro can be separated easily. In plants, "super-glued" inorganic minerals are transformed into "Velcroed" organic minerals. Now, when you eat the plant, your body can break the minerals apart and use their components.

But your body can't use these vital elements if you
don't eat the plants or their produce — vegetables
and fruits.

WELLNESS PRINCIPLE: **Easily accessed plant
                              nutrients are useless to
                              your body until they are
                              eaten.**

Vitamins in plants don't do you much good either
unless you eat them. Plants don't absorb vitamins
from the soil, but plants contain vitamins. It seems
the plants produce them on their own. Clever. Plants
make 'em; you eat 'em. When you eat vegetables and
fruits, you get "first generation" vitamins. You might
say that nature is the only true "drug" store.

What else do vegetables and fruits contain that
you need? Protein.

All living cells contain protein. Protein is made up
of amino acids. So when you have that steak, potato,
and green salad, you get protein from the whole lot —
not just from the steak. If you include a dinner roll or
two, you get more protein.

WELLNESS PRINCIPLE: **You get protein in just
                              about everything you eat.**

We've been talking throughout these chapters
about the perils of eating *too much* protein. Once
again, protein isn't the problem, *too much* protein is
a problem for your body.

COMPLETE PROTEIN

Proteins are made up of amino acids. You may have heard or read that the protein in vegetables and other plant food isn't "complete." This was one of the food-scare forerunners to cholesterol and fat. The incomplete protein concept is that unless you eat meat, poultry, fish, and diary products, you won't get all of the bits and pieces of amino acids you should have. The theme is that vegetables don't have all of the types of amino acids that your body needs. That's another "not quite right" conclusion.

Your body produces some amino acids on its own. These are called *non-essential* amino acids. You don't need to depend on food to provide them. It's not that the amino acids are non-essential to health, they're non-essential in your diet. You don't need to eat them to get them. You come equipped with, or produce, non-essential amino acids. Other amino acids that your body needs are not self-produced. So you must get them from food.

Most vegetables contain most of the essential amino acids your body needs. *Essential amino acids* are those that your body cannot produce naturally on its own. It's *essential* that you consume them. Foods that contain all of the essential amino acids the body needs to make up for those it doesn't produce itself are considered "complete protein" foods.

Foods that are short on essential amino acids are considered "incomplete protein" foods. Celery, lettuce, or turnips, for example, do not have all of the *essential amino acids* your body needs to sustain itself. And fruits contain very few amino acids, although they are big in the vitamin and mineral department. Keep that bit of wisdom in mind if you decide to eat nothing but celery, lettuce, turnips, and fruit for the rest of your life. You won't o.d. on protein, but that may not make much difference because you could suffer from malnutrition — lack of vital life-sustaining nutrients.

When you eat a variety of vegetables at a meal, the essential amino acids of the various vegetables are all schlumped together for your body to use. A little tryptophan here, a bit of threonine there, a tad of lysine and the other essentials from elsewhere, and bingo! — complete protein. Eat two or three or four different vegetables at a meal and you can get all of the essential amino acids.

To give you an idea of how well vegetables can supply your body with essential amino acids, a table showing the amino acid content of some of our more common foods is in the appendix at the back of this book.

WELLNESS PRINCIPLE: **The only protein you miss when you eat a variety of vegetables is animal protein.**

CALLED TO BE A VEGETARIAN?

"If vegetables and fruit are so wonderful," you might ask, "why haven't we evolved to be complete vegetarians?"

The answer to that is simple. Taste. Hamburger, steak, veal cutlets, pork chops, shrimp, crab, turkey, chicken, barbecued ribs, cheese fondue, and the many variations thereof taste good. They are satisfying. They fill us up. They energize us. We like

to eat foods we like. We eat the foods we're
accustomed to eating, and we become accustomed to
eating foods we like. If the foods we like don't
immediately make us sick, chances are we will
continue to eat them. That's the big problem with
dietary animal protein. Most of us like meat, poultry,
and fish. They don't make us sick immediately. But
a steady diet of them can make us "sick" eventually.
However, it takes so long for the "sick" to show up
that we miss the diet connection.

Dyed-in-the-wool meat eaters often complain that
vegetables aren't satisfying. Their fullness factor
suffers. If they don't get a generous helping of meat-
based foods, they aren't satisfied. They get hungry
quickly. That's because their bodies are accustomed
to the "heavier" high-protein diet. Their bodies work
longer and harder to handle all of the debris that
comes along with the meat. So, when they eat meat
and its derivatives, sure 'nuff, their hunger alarm
doesn't clang again for quite a while.

Robust meat-eaters also claim that high-protein
meals energize them. A valid observation. When we
eat meat-based foods, our bodies get very excited
about surviving. When your body is excited about
defending itself, it switches into overdrive to handle
the stress mess. And we interpret the crisis-handling
as "energy."

However, your body adapts to the type of food you
usually eat. If you make a gradual change from
Mostly Meat to Vastly Vegetable, your "fullness
meter" throttles down as your body becomes
accustomed to handling the lighter diet. After a while,
with your new way of eating your "fullness meter"
clicks into "satisfied" and your body clicks into
cruise. But that doesn't mean you'll have less energy

than you did in your heavy meat days. The energy
your body needed to process the animal protein is
now available for you to do other things, like cut the
grass, clean out the attic, climb mountains, play
tennis, and generally work harder and play harder.
Those who have made the switch from Mostly Meat to
Vastly Vegetable have found that as time goes on they
eat less and less meat. Meat slowly loses its appeal.

WELLNESS PRINCIPLE: **In time, Vastly Vegetable
is   satisfaction
guaranteed.**

So, am I advocating that everyone become a
staunch, meat-never-passes-my-lips vegetarian?
NO!
The key to healthful eating is to eat more
vegetables and fruits than meat, poultry, fish, and
their by-products, such as eggs and cheese.
Remember the 70-30 percentages. You don't need to
become a fanatic about your diet. The emotional
stress of holier-than-thou-fanaticism is as hard on
your body as the nutritional stress of dietary animal
protein. And, if you try to convert your friends, it's
equally hard on your social life.

HIGH PROTEIN WITH ROOTS

F ruits and vegetables are probably the best
medicine you can give your body. But, if you
recall, we keep talking about *most* fruits and
vegetables do this and *most* fruits and vegetables do
that. *Most* fruits and vegetables leave an alkaline ash.
Most fruits and vegetables are low in protein. Those

"mosts" are in there for a reason. After all of this "fruits and vegetables are wonderful" business, would you believe that some plant foods leave an acid ash? And some plant foods are high-protein foods.

Indeed, you can over-protein your body with acid ash-producing fruits and vegetables. And the biggest plant-type acid producer is grains.

Grains are the most commonly consumed acid ash-producing plant foods. And do we eat grains! White bread, whole wheat bread, rolls, pancakes, macaroni, spaghetti and other forms of pasta, sweet corn, corn flakes, oatmeal, oat bran, rice, barley, wheat flakes, wheat germ, wheat bran — virtually every meal is spiked with grain in one form or another.

And there are more acid-producing plants. The fruit family has its share. Blueberries, cranberries, currants, plums, and prunes are all acid ash-producers. Those gorgeous, appetizing blueberry muffins that tantalize our taste buds and rev up our saliva glands are packed full of wheat and blueberries — both acid ash-producers. What a bummer!

Much of our popular diet includes many of the aforementioned grains and fruits along with generous portions of meat, poultry, and fish. Small wonder that most of our population is sliding farther and faster down the acid side of the pH scale. And now you know what that means: exhausted organs and systems leading to pain and disease.

Does all of this about acid ash-producing, high-protein grains that are mainstays of our diets put us between the proverbial rock and a hard place when it comes to eating? Hardly a meal (or snack) goes by that we don't munch grains in one form or another.

Are we doomed to have our cells wallow in an increasingly potent sea of acid?

Not at all.

There's an up side to grain protein. Most grains bring along with them quite respectable quantities of all of the essential amino acids plus a few non-essentials (the kind your body generates for itself). Whole wheat flour, for example, offers all of the known essential amino acids.

Grains may leave an acid ash, but they also leave more neutralizing minerals than do meats. These neutralizing minerals help to buffer the acid left in the body. But they can't do the whole job. That's why strict vegetarians who eat a lot of grains can become sick from an overly acid internal environment just as meat-eaters can.

WELLNESS PRINCIPLE: **Acidosis is not limited to meat-eaters.**

To keep their bodies on an even pH level, vegetarians must make sure they balance their grain intake with plenty of alkaline ash-producing vegetables and fruits. As with most things in life, moderation in grain consumption is the key.

A GREAT INTERNAL BALANCING ACT

Your body works toward balance — equilibrium. If your body is cold, it shivers to warm itself up. If it's hot, it perspires to cool itself off. If it's too acid, it calls on backup systems to neutralize it. If it's too alkaline, it incites internal activity that produces acid. Balance is good.

But, here's an out-of-balance situation that may be new to you. It's related to the types of food you eat — contractive and expansive foods.

The terms "contractive" and "expansive" aren't far-out words, but we don't often hear them applied to foods.

"Contractive," as it relates to foods, refers to a drawing in, squeezing, or limiting effect the foods have on the body. We're not talking about reducing body size. We're talking about an internal tightening or restricting — up-tightness. "Expansive" relates to opening out, blossoming, or inflating. Again, not body size — it's an internal effect. Both expansive and contractive foods can stress your body and affect your mental attitude.

WELLNESS PRINCIPLE: **Highly contractive or highly expansive foods mean a highly stressed body.**

In general, acidifying foods are contractive. They lead to an up-tight attitude. Similarly, in general, alkalizing foods are expansive foods that promote a loose, laid-back, possibly spacy outlook. A few foods, however, are neither highly expansive nor highly contractive; they're neutral.

Neutral foods are least-stress foods. The most neutral of all foods is nature's absolute best get-this-small-person-off-to-a-good-start food — mother's milk. But mother's milk is a short-term food for infants. For toddlers through adults, the foods that put the least stress on the body are those closest to neutral. Least-stress foods on the contractive side are grains, nuts, seeds, and beans. Least-stress foods on the expansive side are vegetables and fruits.

Graphically it looks like the following diagram. The Most Contractive and Most Expansive are at the top of each list descending to Least Contractive and Least Expansive at the bottom.

CONTRACTIVE AND EXPANSIVE FOODS

Very Contractive   **Very Expansive**

H   I   G   H   S   T   R   E   S   S

	Drugs
	Liquor
	Beer
Salt	Wine
Red Meat	Sugar
Fowl	Syrups
Eggs	Chocolate
Fish	Coffee
Chicken	Tea
Butter	Fruit Juice

L   O   W   S   T   R   E   S   S

Slightly Contractive   **Slightly Expansive**

Beans	
Seeds	
Nuts	Fruits
Grains	Vegetables

On this graphic, the higher the food in the list, the more expansive or contractive it is. Fruits and vegetables, at the bottom of the expansive list, are the least expansive. They are "slightly expansive."

Increasingly expansive are fruit juice, tea, coffee, chocolate, syrups (honey and molasses), sugar, wine, beer, liquor, and the most expansive of all, prescription, over-the-counter, and recreational (usually illegal) drugs.

On the contractive side, at the bottom, grains, nuts, seeds, and beans are "slightly contractive." Increasingly contractive are butter, chicken, fish, eggs, fowl, red meat, and the top contractor, salt. These are the diet mainstays of the ardent meat-eaters. Contractive foods are essentially acid-producing foods, and acid-producing foods are essentially contractive foods.

Your body achieves a level of balance, even if the foods you eat are either mostly contractive or mostly expansive. The balancing results may show up in your personality. A predominantly contractive personality expresses itself in various forms of quick temper, explosiveness, or aggression. If not outright physical aggression, it may be masked as constant nervousness, physical overactivity, or verbal overactivity. Contractive personalities are the "don't just sit there, do something" folks. Always busy, always over scheduled, often flying off the handle, foot tappers. Contractive persons, and personalities, usually eat a lot of meat and top it off with salt and more salt. You know the kind — when they sit down to eat, the first thing they do is pick up the salt shaker and have at it. Salt first, taste later is their motto. Table salt is the most highly contractive ingredient of all. And your body can't even put it to good use!

**WELLNESS PRINCIPLE: A contractive personality is a
hallmark of an overly acid
body.**

A predominantly expansive personality is casual,
laid-back, unable to concentrate, not "grounded," and
minimally motivated, perhaps to the extent of being
the proverbial ne'er-do-well. Despite their laid-
backness, expansive personality people tend to be
worriers. They don't fidget. They are the "don't just do
something, sit there and fret" advocates. Some
overzealous vegetarians can become so expansive
they appear to be on "cloud nine" — barely in touch
with reality.

Drugs, alcohol, chocolate, coffee, tea, and fruit
juices are big favorites of the expansives. The most
expansive substances we can put into our bodies are
drugs. But items that appear lower on the expansive
list can have "drug-like" effects and also leave their
mark on the personality.

Fruit juice? That's far from being a drug.

Fruits themselves are slightly expansive. Fruit
juice is a concentrated form of fruit, therefore, it is a
little more expansive than whole fruit. You can drink
a lot more fruit in juice form than you can eat in
whole form. You can o.d. on fruit juice. My clinical
experience shows that drinking large quantities of
fruit juice can have a "tranquilizing" effect on adults.
However, as with many other "drugs," large quantities
of fruit juice can have just the opposite effect on
children. Instead of calming them down, it revs them
up. One symptom is what might be termed "the
orange juice cough." This is a persistent, non-
productive cough. No phlegm, just cough.

WELLNESS PRINCIPLE: Your diet affects more than how your body works, it affects how you work.

Few of us limit our diets exclusively to only contractive or only expansive foods. Most. meals contain some of both. Consequently, most of us don't exhibit the dramatic personality types of extreme aggression or extreme spaciness. We're more likely to be moderate in our contractive or expansive personality displays. We may be moderately aggressive — impatient, bossy, negative, overly critical of others, generally at odds with the world but able to function well enough. Or we may be moderately spacy — disorganized, easily distracted, have trouble following a project through to completion, worry a lot, generally have an outwardly easy-going outlook, but grounded enough to do those things that ought to be done.

Now, how's that for laying it on the line. I'm not telling you that vegetables and fruits are the answer to all of life's problems. I'm telling you that you need to eat plant food in order to give your body the nutrients it needs to keep your internal environment a neat place for your cells to live. Most Americans eat some fruits and vegetables. However, all too many of us don't eat enough. Your body is geared to handle vegetables and fruits. And, even if they aren't your favorite foods now, they will climb on your "Gee, that's pretty good" list when your body finds out what it has been missing.

OVERCOMING CREEPING ACIDOSIS

So, what have we learned about vegetables and fruits?

The most important thing is that vegetables and fruits supply most of the neutralizing ingredients your body needs. That's the biggie concept. Without an adequate supply of alkaline ash-producing foods, your body will eventually suffer from acidosis. You don't just develop acidosis, you suffer from it. Creeping acidosis leads to all manner of aches, pains, and debilitating diseases that we usually attribute to bad luck or heredity.

The first line of defense against creeping acidosis is a generous supply of vegetables and fruits in your diet. When you provide the materials your body needs to neutralize acid and replenish your alkaline reserve, your body doesn't have to work overtime just to survive your diet. And remember, your body will do everything and anything necessary to survive this instant.

> **WELLNESS PRINCIPLE:** A proper diet helps keep your body from working itself to death just to survive.

You don't need to become a vegetarian to be healthy or keep your internal acid level under control. Many vegetarians have the same problem with acid that meat-eaters do. They over acidify their bodies. But instead of overacidifying on meat, vegetarians overacidify on acid ash-producing grains. And too much acid is too much acid no matter where it comes from.

The best thing for your body is to make sure you eat more alkaline ash-producing foods than you do acid ash-producing foods. Again, the ideal percentage is about 70% alkaline ash, and 30% acid ash. If you are big into meat at every meal now, the 70-30 ratio is a goal you work toward — slowly. You don't go from 95% acid ash-producing to 25% overnight. Well, you can. But you won't like the short-term results. You'll be sick, sick, sick. Your body isn't ready to make a big transition quickly. Remember those enzymes? Changing your diet really means re-tooling your enzymes. And that doesn't happen overnight.

If you suspect that your body may be too acid for its own good, don't jump onto the I'll-eat-only-fruits-and-vegetables horse too quickly. It'll throw you for sure.

The best method of introducing more vegetables into your diet is just that. Introduce them one serving at a time — don't adopt the whole lot all at once. After a few days, introduce a second serving. A few days later, add some more. But if you're really acid, stay away from raw fresh fruit until your body is ready to handle it.

Farther along in this book, you'll find a more detailed schedule for upgrading your health-reducing diet to a diet that is health-producing.

In the meantime, let's take a trip through an overly acid body to see how it copes to survive.

CHAPTER 6

THE ROCKY ROAD TO GALLSTONES

We have seen that blood pH must stay between 7.35 and 7.45. That's on the alkaline side of neutral pH 7.0. However, when acid ash foods constantly push the pH of the internal environment to the acid side, the body must respond to correct the situation. It's a "Save the blood!" campaign that's waged without thought by either you or your body.

Blood is only one fluid in the body. There are others inside and outside the cells. Some of those fluids have interesting pH ranges that are considered "normal." For example:

Liver bile	pH 7.8 - 8.6	(Slightly alkaline to
Pancreatic fluid	pH 7.2 - 8.6	mildly alkaline)
Gallbladder bile	pH 4.5 - 8.5	(Strong acid for the body
Urine	pH 4.5 - 8.4	to mildly alkaline)
Stomach fluids	pH 1.0 - 3.0	(Really strong acid)
Saliva	pH 6.5 - 7.45	(Slightly acid to slightly alkaline)

These ranges are interesting because we know that slight changes in pH numbers can mean big changes in acidity or alkalinity. They are also interesting because we know that the body works best when it is slightly alkaline. Why, then, would there be so much backing and forthing from acid to alkaline of essential fluids? Gallbladder bile, for example. At pH 4.5, gallbladder bile is quite acid; at pH 8.5, it's mildly alkaline. That's a big pH swing.

Here's a clue: There's a difference between "normal" and "necessary." The fluid values are considered "normal." As we shall see, pH fluctuations from one extreme to another are more than "normal," they are "necessary" for survival.

WELLNESS PRINCIPLE: "Necessary" may not be "normal."

To shed some light on the mystery of the wide-ranging pH, join me on a short "virtual reality" trip through the digestive system. With the help of our imaginations, we shrink ourselves down to wander-through-the-body-size. We'll take along a rough sketch of the inner territory to help us identify some land marks. Now, with trusty imaginary pH meter and reference book in hand, we'll see if we can find out what's behind such dramatic fluctuations in the pH of some of our vital fluids. Into the mouth we go.

Here we are in the Grand Cavern, slipping and sliding on a saliva covered tongue surrounded by great white mountains. The perfect place for our first pH measurement. We already know what to expect — we passed the list just a couple of paragraphs ago. The pH "normal" for saliva hovers between slightly acid 6.5 and slightly alkaline 7.45. But our pH meter shows the saliva here is pH 5.8. The environment is a little more acid than "normal." That's strange. That's not the ideal working environment for the saliva enzyme ptyalin that starts the digestion process with a slight nudge.

Ptyalin works best in a pH environment of 7.0 or above. Why would an enzyme be placed in an inhospitable environment to do its job? Since the characteristics of ptyalin are fixed but the environment isn't, a better question is, why is the saliva pH so low? It can't be a problem with the pH meter; imaginary instruments are always accurate. And the body never does anything just for kicks. There must be a good reason why the saliva is more acid than "normal." We'll move on to see if we can solve this mystery.

Over tongue and into the throat, we pick up peristaltic waves of the esophagus and surf into the stomach. We don't need instruments to tell us that this is a strong acid environment. Yuck! The pH meter registers 2.0. That's acid. Hydrochloric acid is being pumped from cells of the walls. There's a lot of recently eaten high-protein food in here. Look at the way the food is arranged. It lines the walls in layers. Food doesn't just land in a heap all jumbled together. It's in layers. First in, first nestled against the walls.

And enzymes. There are enzymes that help in the digestion process. How can enzymes function in an environment as acid as this?

According to our reference book, pepsin is one of the main enzymes in the stomach. Pepsin works in a pH 2.0 to 3.0 environment. So this is a great working environment for pepsin. Pepsin begins the digestion of proteins. With all of the protein in here, the pepsin has its work cut out for it. The atmosphere is really

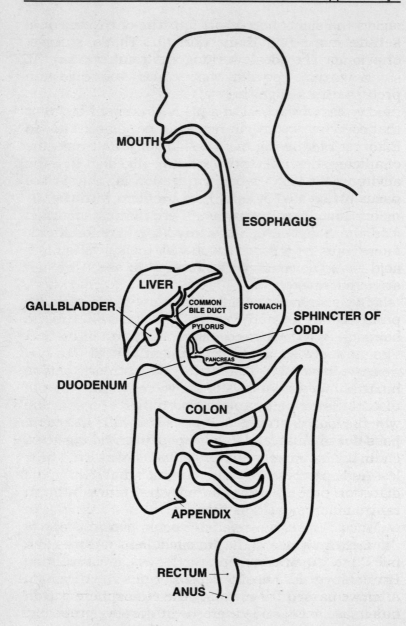

acid — efficient for breaking down food, but not nice. Let's get out of here. Over there, through the pylorus, or pyloric valve if you prefer, and into the duodenum.

Now, this is what you call acid relief. It's still pretty acid, but there's a lot of mucus. Alkaline mucus everywhere. The mucus is coming from glands that cover the walls of the duodenum. They are called Brunner's glands. Lots of Brunner's glands and lots of alkaline mucus. Our reference book says that the acidity of the duodenum depends on whether or not partially digested food is being pumped through the pylorus into the duodenum. This partially digested food is called chyme (pronounced kime). When chyme moves into the duodenum, the atmosphere is pretty acid. When there's no food coming through, the atmosphere is slightly alkaline. What do you know, "slightly alkaline" again. Right now, with the stomach pumping out a steady stream of chyme, it's hard to believe that this place could ever be slightly alkaline. Time to move on. There's a lot more to see.

As we slog our way through the mucus-chyme mixture, we pass by a narrow opening in the duodenal wall. Fluid is flowing from the opening which is labeled "To Common Bile Duct." After we pass the opening, the atmosphere and landscape change. All of a sudden our pH meter shows there is less acid. And we notice there are fewer Brunner's glands. The pH here is in the more moderate 5.5 range. Much more pleasant. That's a quick change in weather. Let's stop and think about this.

Before we arrived at the opening to the common bile duct, the atmosphere was very acid and a lot of Brunner's glands were pumping out a lot of mucus. After we passed the opening, the atmosphere wasn't quite as acid and there were fewer protective

Brunner's glands to produce mucus. That makes sense. If the atmosphere is less acid, fewer Brunner's glands and less mucus are needed. But why did the atmosphere improve? And why is it still acid at all? We'll move out of the path of the food that's being digested and see if we can find out what caused the change in the climate. We'll take a side trip up the common bile duct.

The entrance to the duct is pretty tight for us to slither through. However, the fluids that come down the duct every day have no problem as long as the way is clear. As we swim upstream we notice that the fluid mixture is slightly acid. After a very short swim, we come to a fork in the channel. Imaginary directional signs tell us that the right fork leads to

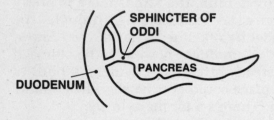

the pancreas. Off to the left is the road to the gallbladder and liver. We've been swimming in a fluid mixture coming from the pancreas, gallbladder, and liver. Let's explore the pancreas first.

As we slip through the sphincter of Oddi "gate" to the pancreatic duct there's a definite improvement in the atmosphere. We're in a pH 7.2 to 8.6 environment. Clear fluid resembling saliva streams from the pancreas — about a quart a day. Our reference book tells us that the pancreas is a bee hive of activity. Internally, it produces insulin that is delivered directly to the blood. The fluid we're navigating is pancreatic fluid that is produced externally and gushes down the pancreatic duct.

Pancreatic fluid contains three major enzymes that are programmed to work in a comfortable alkaline environment of pH 7.5 to 8.2. The enzyme protease works on protein, lipase works on fats, and carbohydrase works on carbohydrates. That makes sense. Protein, fat, and carbohydrate are the three types of foods we need in a well-balanced diet.

In addition to the enzymes, there's a lot of pH 8.0 sodium bicarbonate. Nice weather in here. Great working conditions for the resident enzymes. It's off to the left fork now to see what's going on in there.

The atmosphere in the duct that goes to the liver is back on the acid side again. A short way up this duct we come to another opening in the wall. It's labeled "To the Gallbladder." This place is beginning to take on an Alice in Wonderland atmosphere. We almost expect to see the white rabbit come scurrying along our path.

As we pass the entrance to the gallbladder headed toward the liver, we're in normal liver bile. The pH here is between 7.8 and 8.6.

That's interesting. The "weather" changes every time we go through an opening. The fluids from the openings we've encountered along the way have a major effect on the atmosphere of the surrounding countryside. First, we left the strong acid environment of the stomach and went into weaker acid in the duodenum. Then we passed by the opening to the common bile duct and there was even less acid. The fluid was slightly acid in the common bile duct. And when we went through the sphincter of Oddi to get to the pancreas, we encountered alkalinity in the pancreatic duct. In the common bile duct on the way to the gallbladder and liver, we found fairly strong acid. Now, just by moving "upstream" from the opening to the gallbladder we're in very comfortable alkali. That's odd. Why isn't the whole area slightly alkaline? What happened to the "sightly alkaline" internal environment the body works toward?

We'll see if we can figure this out. Our reference book says that gallbladder bile can be as low as pH 4.5 and as high as pH 8.6. But the gallbladder stores liver bile. And liver bile checks in at a comfortable pH 7.8 to 8.5. If the gallbladder is just *storing* liver bile, how could it possibly have a pH as low as 4.5? There must be a good reason. The situation may seem strange, but the body never does anything stupid or wrong. This bears further investigation. C'mon. Into the gallbladder to see what's going on.

The first thing we notice is the climate — zesty! The pH has dropped to a pungent 5.5. Maybe the gallbladder is an acid-producing organ like the stomach. But the reference book doesn't say anything about the gallbladder *producing* acid. It says the pH of the contents of the gallbladder can be as low as 4.5, but it doesn't say how it gets that acid.

So, if the gallbladder doesn't produce acid, where is the acid coming from? Certainly not from the liver. The liver produces bile with a pH of 7.8 to 8.6 — definitely alkaline.

Our reference book also tells us that gallbladder bile is thicker than liver bile. Can't argue about that. The stuff in here borders on being lumpy sludge. The reference book says that gallbladder bile is concentrated. Can't argue about that either. It's obviously more concentrated than liver bile. Maybe that's why it's more acid.

Let's sit down on one of these little lumps and examine this situation.

"Concentrate" means to increase the strength of a fluid by evaporation. Concentrating an alkaline substance shouldn't make it more acid. The substance possesses the same properties; it just loses water. Kind of like concentrated orange juice. If concentration alters the pH of an alkaline fluid, it should make it more alkaline, not acid. So concentration can't be the reason for the acidity. Something else is going on. Let's see. What else is in bile?

Electrolytes!

Alkaline liver bile stored in the gallbladder contains electrolytes. Electrolytes, such as sodium, potassium, and chloride salts, play an important part in conducting internal electric currents. (Of course you realize that we are really bundles of energy.)

Alkaline liver bile is well-stocked with electrolytes when it is stored in the gallbladder. These electrolytes are then reabsorbed from the gallbladder and put back into the bloodstream. That's why the bile is concentrated. And that's why the bile is acid. Sodium and other neutralizing minerals have been reabsorbed from the liver bile and put into the bloodstream.

But, why would sodium and other electrolytes be taken out of liver bile when liver bile should be alkaline? The body doesn't do foolish things. There must be a very good reason. Could it have something to do with the type of foods that have coursed through this body? If the contents of the stomach and duodenum are an indication of this person's diet, this body has been dealing with a lot of dietary protein. The sodium in the liver bile is needed to perform functions more important to survival than keeping bile alkaline and fluid.

Sodium reabsorption is a perfectly normal function of the body. The problem seems to be the quantity of sodium that's reabsorbed. Instead of most of it staying in the bile, great amounts are reabsorbed into the bloodstream to be used to meet more important needs, such as neutralizing blood and urine. When sodium and other electrolytes are reabsorbed into the bloodstream they are available to neutralize acids from excess protein. As a result, the bile in the gallbladder becomes more acid and concentrated. The body isn't doing anything it wasn't designed to do. Neutralizing elements are supposed to be taken from gallbladder bile. But not so many that the bile becomes overly thick, acid, and lumpy.

We've been so preoccupied with the pH and thickness of the sludgy fluid here in the gallbladder that we haven't paid any attention to the lumps. They look like pebbles, rocks, and boulders.

They're gallstones! And we've been using one for our study bench.

We seem to have stumbled onto something significant here. According to our reference book, the principal ingredient in gallstones is cholesterol. Cholesterol isn't very soluble in water. It needs bile salts and other substances to help break it down. When bile is concentrated, the bile salts are also concentrated to keep the cholesterol liquid. However, this particular body is woefully short of the sodium the gallbladder needs for liquid bile salts. Neutralizing minerals are in short supply throughout the body. They are being used where they are needed for survival. The blood must be kept slightly alkaline — it's a matter of life or death.

The body, in its infinite wisdom, will take all the neutralizing minerals it needs to keep the blood in

slightly alkaline survival range. We can't survive with
"acid blood." We can survive with gallstones. They
just hurt and plug up ducts.

Remember, the body doesn't worry about the
future. It doesn't think and it doesn't plan. The body
performs perfectly to survive conditions of the
moment. It doesn't consider future consequences of
present survival activities. It is concerned with
current situations only. Gallstones are
inconsequential consequences of past survival
tactics.

With bile salts in short supply, cholesterol has
accumulated and "solidified." Now, it is "stones." And
with the number of stones in this gallbladder, very
likely the gallbladder owner is in major pain and
distress and getting ready to have the offending organ
removed.

Will that help?

Yes, indeed. It will help the symptoms. But
gallbladder removal in itself won't help the underlying
cause of the symptoms. A major change of diet and
lifestyle is needed to get at the cause. After the
gallbladder is gone, unless the body receives
generous supplies of usable neutralizing minerals
each day, it will still be subjected to non-stop acid
attacks. In time, other symptoms will show up
someplace else. But, of course, the symptoms will be
so far removed from the dinner table that the
association will still be missed.

"But," you respond, "the people I know who have
had their gallbladder removed can eat anything they
want and they feel great!"

Correct! They do feel great. No more "gallbladder
attacks." No more discomfort after eating. No more
diet restrictions. All seems right with the world. But

now you can see that their problem hasn't been
solved. It's just been shifted, but they don't know it
yet.

You can see why removing the gallbladder
removes symptoms. With the gallbladder gone, only
alkaline liver bile and alkaline pancreatic fluids flow
into the duodenum. This means that the chyme is
buffered (neutralized) from really acid to pleasantly
alkaline. No acid bile pain, no burn. However,
without the gallbladder, the body can't reclaim the
sodium and other goodies from the liver bile. The
sodium supply is already overtaxed. Cut out the
gallbladder and one of the body's major suppliers of
neutralizing minerals goes with it. With one of the
major suppliers gone, the body will call on other
minerals to keep the acid level under control. And
here we are back at osteoporosis.

Wow! Our imaginary trip through part of the
digestive system turned out to be more than we
bargained for. What have we learned?

For one thing, we learned why normally alkaline
saliva was acid at the beginning of this imaginary
trip. Acid saliva may be an indicator of sodium
shortfall in the body. (Acid saliva can also be an
indicator of emotional override, but that's another
book.) You can get along with acid saliva when the
body is low on alkalizing minerals. It's not the best
situation, but it beats acid blood.

We've also learned that the pH of gallbladder bile
depends on the general availability of neutralizing
minerals throughout the body. When the general
store is short of the necessary minerals, more
minerals are taken from gallbladder bile. And without
enough minerals to keep the bile fluid, gallstones
form.

And there's more.

When gallbladder bile becomes acid, it mixes with alkaline liver bile and pancreatic fluid in the common bile duct. When strong acid is mixed with moderate alkaline, the end result is slight acidity. Fluid flowing from the common bile duct into the duodenum is supposed to be alkaline to neutralize acid chyme. But because the gallbladder fluid is acid, the pancreatic/gallbladder fluid emptying into the duodenum is slightly acid. When you dump "slightly acid" into "strong acid," you get more acid. That's very significant!

Recall how the landscape of the duodenum changed after we passed the opening to the common bile duct. Fewer Brunner's glands dotted the walls and less mucus was present. That's a great arrangement if the fluid from the common bile duct is alkaline. It's not so great if the fluid coming from the common bile duct is acid. At that point in the digestive tract, delicate tissue isn't protected against acid. So what happens to this delicate tissue when it is constantly washed with acid? It gets burned.

Good Golly, Miss Molly! Do you realize what that means? Most of those people who are running around suffering with "duodenal ulcers" are actually suffering from "acid bile burn." It's not acid from the stomach that's causing the problem — it's acid fluid (that should be alkaline) from the common bile duct.

That's enough excitement for one trip. Let's get out of here, "reinflate" ourselves, and ponder some of our discoveries.

Perhaps the biggest lesson we learned (or reinforced) is that health and disease are whole-body conditions. The rocky road to gallstones is a whole-body problem. Gallstones aren't the problem. The problem is too much protein constantly coming down the pike. The body's reserve of neutralizing minerals has been drained. The body is operating in survival mode just to keep the internal environment a decent place for the cells to live.

Most people have no problem accepting the connection between diet and gallbladder problems. But as we have seen, the problem isn't the effect diet has on the gallbladder; it's the effect diet has on the whole body. The gallbladder is part of the interconnected, internal network of organs and systems. The gallbladder is merely one example of how a particular organ and a particular pattern of symptoms indicate a "sick body." It's an alkaline reserve problem. And since the availability of alkaline reserve minerals affects the entire body, it's a body problem!

All of the body's intricate parts and systems are superbly designed, engineered, and interrelated. Even when one particular organ or system is the focal point of a disease, the whole-body was sick before specific symptoms showed up in any one organ. The good news is that your body provides you with tell-tale signs that something is amiss even before painful, debilitating symptoms appear and become disease. That's the next chapter.

CHAPTER 7

THE ENERGY DRAIN

HEALTH AND DISEASE ARE THOUGHTLESS

Here we are in the most affluent, technologically advanced country on earth yet great numbers of us can tic off lengthy laundry lists of personal ills. Chronic fatigue. Diabetes. Osteoporosis. Arthritis. Kidney disease. Liver disease. Heart disease. Pick-an-organ disease. Allergies. Headaches. Back pain. Muscle pain. Shoulder, knee, elbow, or other joint pain. The combinations of aches and pains are endless. Being "tired" is a national pastime.

> **WELLNESS PRINCIPLE:** If we're so rich and smart, how come we're so sick and tired?

We get sick when we push our bodies' survival skills to extremes just to handle the consequences of our choices and actions. Pain and disease are survival effects. You're not sick because you have diabetes or whatever. You have diabetes or whatever because you're sick. Pain and disease certainly appear to be results of the body doing something "wrong." But they're not. Pain and disease are results of the body surviving to the point of exhaustion. Energy that should be used to accomplish your daily activities is being used to keep your body alive. Survival is more important than accomplishment.

The body doesn't do "wrong." As long as the body functions at all, it functions perfectly, and it functions only to survive. Perfect internal survival functions don't require any thought on your part. When you exert yourself, you don't need to think about raising your heart rate or your blood pressure. Your body doesn't wait for you to become concerned that your blood pH is stretching the outer limits before it begins to respond. Your sympathetic nervous system doesn't wait for detailed instructions on when and how to handle a threatening situation. The thousands of internal adjustments your body constantly makes are all carried out without your conscious help. And they're done just right. They are perfect for survival. Always.

Everything the body does is correct to survive the conditions and stimuli of the moment. Everything it has ever done was to survive that moment. If it hadn't functioned in precisely the right way to survive each moment of the past, it would have stopped functioning. That means dead. Whatever the body is doing or has done is a survival tactic. We may call the symptoms brought about by persistent, repetitive survival functions "disease." As far as the body is concerned it's called "moment-to-moment survival."

WELLNESS PRINCIPLE: The body doesn't do health or disease; it does survival.

You either survive or die. When you realize that the body responds only to survive, you realize that even responses that we classify as disease are survival responses. Your disease is the "cure" for the effects of your inappropriate choices and actions. That's a difficult concept for many people to accept, especially if they are in pain or unable to move easily and do the things they used to do.

> **WELLNESS PRINCIPLE: Your comfort and ease of movement are not survival concerns.**

Again, your body doesn't think or plan for the future. You do that with your conscious mind. Physiological responses aren't products of your conscious mind. They are often *influenced* by your conscious mind, but they aren't *directed* by your conscious mind. You might include thanks for that when you acknowledge your many gifts and graces. Can you imagine what your life would be like if you had to think consciously about keeping your heart beating, your pancreas functioning, your intestines undulating, and the other thousands of internal processes going — and going in synch? The individual parts and systems of your body are not independent. They work together, without you prompting them, for survival of the whole. So if your pancreas, liver, heart, or kidneys have a problem, you have a whole-body problem.

The concept of whole-body survival as opposed to single-organ disease is repeated in various forms throughout this book. That's because it is so important. We might say that this concept is the foundation for understanding why you are, or are not, as healthy as you would like to be.

Disease doesn't strike. Disease develops. It develops as the body adapts continuously to survive particular threatening conditions. For example, the excess acid from high protein foods that we've been talking about. If the body must adapt constantly to handle this excess acid, two things happen. One, the availability of alkalizing minerals from the alkaline reserve is greatly reduced, and, two, backup systems that were designed for emergency-service-only must work in high gear constantly. The results of these conditions: (1) Some internal functions are short-changed — neutralizing minerals must be scavenged from other sources, such as the bones, and (2) internal emergency organs and systems are pushed beyond their capacity and eventually become exhausted. Now it's called disease.

When organs and systems become exhausted, disease is the next step. Usually, the disease affects the "weakest link." The particular disease that develops depends on which organ or system has a hereditary tendency to "weakness" and/or has been hardest hit by what you have been doing to keep your body in hyper-survival mode. Your body is surviving all the time. When you make choices that keep one area on red-alert constantly, that area gets tired. The process generally goes on for so long that you don't associate the cause with the effect. The cause is the choices you make that your body must survive. The effect is what you interpret as disease. Without the survival processes that lead to the effects you interpret as disease, you wouldn't be around long enough to get sick.

WELLNESS PRINCIPLE: Disease is a solution to a problem.

DISEASE — IT FOLLOWS

Disease is a symptom of exhaustion. Organs and systems can become exhausted when they must function either in an inhospitable environment, or function non-stop. And if they are subjected to both crummy environment and no vacation, you've inflicted a double whammy on your body.

No system or organ of the body is designed to function at full-speed without rest. Every part of your body needs rest. Your heart rests between beats. Your digestive organs and systems rest between feedings. But even without rest, they'll keep going as long as possible to survive. That's exhausting. When they're exhausted, they can't function as well as you would like. Eventually, symptoms develop.

Symptoms aren't "things." And symptoms aren't really "symptoms" until you know about them. For example, your blood pressure can launch into stellar space without you realizing it. But high blood pressure doesn't qualify as hypertension or a "symptom" until it is detected and labeled as such, or you have a stroke or heart attack. That's why you can go into a doctor's office for a check-up feeling great and come out "sick." Your internal processes don't change significantly in the few hours you are there, but your attitude and view of the future certainly can. Symptoms are your conscious interpretation of something that's going on in your body that produces effects you don't like. You don't often hear a friend complain that he or she is suffering symptoms of severe, unremitting health and energy. Symptoms are your clue that an organ or system has been overworked in its effort to survive. Exhaustion has set in. And it's the symptoms of exhaustion that we label as a particular disease.

If you get the impression that I'm stressing the exhaustion-symptom-disease relationship, you're right. Locking on to a firm grasp of this concept may be vital to your future health. Physiological exhaustion leads to disease! And inappropriate choices in the six essential areas (eating, drinking, resting, exercising, breathing, and thinking) lead to physiological exhaustion.

WELLNESS PRINCIPLE: We set ourselves up for health or disease.

For too long we have given medical doctors the responsibility for our health. And what happens? Most of us do pretty much what we want to do in the area of the six essentials, then when symptoms start to show up, we go to the doctor to "get fixed." The doctor does his or her best, and we usually feel better. But if we don't feel better or we don't like the results, we sue. Doesn't make sense, does it? We abuse our bodies, go to the doctor to "get fixed," keep on doing what we were doing to get in the predicament in the first place, then become upset when the "fixing" doesn't hold.

Who is responsible for your health?

Doctors can generally help to relieve symptoms, but they aren't responsible for monitoring our thoughts and actions to keep us healthy. We need to understand that each of us individually is responsible for our personal health. It's up to us, as responsible adults, to give our bodies the same consideration we give our valuable possessions.

We don't put leaded fuel in a car that is engineered to use unleaded. But we think nothing about fueling our alkaline designed bodies with too much acid-producing protein.

We don't keep calling 911 because the house might catch fire sometime in the nebulous future. But many people keep themselves primed for a possible emergency all day every day. That's called worry or anxiety.

We take responsibility for our own health when we make sure the fuel and other stimuli we put into our bodies are the kinds that our bodies can use to the best advantage. When we do this, our bodies don't become exhausted, we're not troubled with unpleasant symptoms, and disease doesn't gain a foothold.

WELLNESS PRINCIPLE: Your   health   is   your responsibility.

Diet is a big contributor to exhaustion, symptoms, and disease. A body that is flooded daily with acid from too much protein works constantly to overcome the excess acidity. The body can do that — for survival. However, enough is enough. You're designed to walk and talk and run and climb stairs. But if you do all or any of those day and night, year after year, you're going to get a little tired. Your acid fighting functions can be affected the same way.

When you overload your body with acid ash foods day in and day out, your body must continuously drum up standard and alternative methods of keeping your body alkaline. In time, not only are systems and organs exhausted, but your supply of available alkaline reserve minerals is exhausted. The

end result is symptoms of disease. And you may not
realize that the disease symptoms are even remotely
connected with diet or other choices you make in the
six essential areas of life. So instead of complaining
about disease, be thankful that your body can adapt
to keep you alive despite your eating and lifestyle
indiscretions.

> **WELLNESS PRINCIPLE: Health is more than the
> absence of symptoms.**

SUBTLE SYMPTOMS

P ain is the most obvious symptom of disease or
"trouble" in your body. However, not all
symptoms are painful. Symptoms of acidosis don't
appear suddenly. They, like the acidosis itself, "creep
up" — creeping acidosis. Creeping acidosis is
different from the acidosis that you will experience
when you take the pH challenge described in the next
chapter. That's when you intentionally flood your
body with high-protein food for a couple of days and
raise your internal acid level quickly. However, that's
a temporary surge of acid. The kind of acidosis we're
talking about here comes from months and years of
day-after-day high-protein intake. This is the diet
regimen that strains your alkaline reserve and
backup systems. And this is the diet regimen that is
the *cause* of much of the pain and misery that show
up in doctors' offices.

> **WELLNESS PRINCIPLE: Acidosis doesn't strike — it
> "creeps up."**

However, before you reach crisis level acidosis, your infinitely intelligent body often provides pre-pain warning signs that it is overly acid. These pre-pain signs, like road signs in a foreign language, are easily ignored if you don't know how to read them. One of the most important early indicators of excess acidosis is the inability to sleep six to seven hours straight without waking up.

In 1921, Hasker Kritzer, MD, offered a list of nine symptoms of acidosis. These symptoms are so mild and so commonplace that it's hard to think of them as legitimate "symptoms." They don't hurt or interfere with the day's activities. They appear to be more personality traits than symptoms. In fact, you may recognize these symptoms in your family members, friends, spouse, children, or even yourself. Here is a summary of Dr. Kritzer's 75-year old observations.

Symptoms of Acidosis

1. Exaggerated sense of well-being — belief that he/she is perfectly healthy.
2. Overly ambitious — very restless.
3. Increasingly irritable and ill-tempered — disagreeable to family and friends.
4. Difficult to please — fault-finder.
5. Pessimist — sees only the down side of every situation.
6. Restless sleeper.
7. Wakes up tired in the morning — needs coffee, and perhaps a cigarette, to start the day.
8. Becomes increasingly fatigued — physical symptoms begin to appear.
9. Begins to have muscle weakness or cramps — calcium loss in bone not as obvious.

That's scary. It's a personality profile of huge numbers of people in this country. But then, huge numbers of people in this country follow diets that make them prime candidates for acidosis.

Many of the symptoms of acidosis are more obvious to others than to the symptom bearer. Irritability, pessimism, and fault-finding send large ripples through social and business relationships. However, more personal signs and symptoms can give earlier warnings of creeping acidosis. Diarrhea, constipation, a cold. Even not being hungry for days but continuing to eat every meal anyway. Any major change in the way you feel or the way your body is functioning indicates that your body is seeking balance of some sort.

The common cold is more than just annoying. It is one of your body's methods of cleaning itself from the inside. Scientists can do test tube searches of the germ world from now until forever to find the cause of the common cold and still come up empty-handed. The cause of the common cold isn't germs. Germs are with us all the time. The cause of most colds is toxicity that lowers the resistance of the body. The runny nose, coughing, and sneezing symptoms of a cold are the body's way of cleansing itself of excess toxins. This cleansing can return the body to a more normal state. Have you ever noticed how good you feel after you have had a cold?

Flu falls into the same category. If flu germs were the sole cause of flu epidemics, everyone would get it. But not everyone does. Even in a family that lives together, some get the flu, others don't. You get the flu when your body is working to survive serious threats, like toxic acidosis. Toxicity lowers resistance of the body, and lowered resistance is the welcome mat for germs.

Symptoms of colds and flu usually aren't subtle; they're miserable. Colds and flu are signs that the body is toxic, needs cleaning, and is exhausted. Its resources for survival are being taxed. Resistance has plummeted.

But colds and flu serve a useful purpose. They are cleansing processes. Colds and flu are solutions to the overly toxic internal environment. The body is cleaning itself out. Granted, the side effects of a cold or flu are unpleasant — runny nose, watery eyes, cough, achy muscles and joints, and a general feeling of the blahs. In the process of all of this physiological upheaval, undesirables are washed from the internal environment. And if the internal mess has really gotten out of hand with more mess than mere washing will handle, the internal temperature rises enough to "burn up" unwanted waste materials — we call that a "fever."

WELLNESS PRINCIPLE: You don't "catch" colds or flu; you earn them.

You can detect subtle indicators of acidosis by doing the Fist-, Sniff-, and Stiff-tests that were introduced in Chapter 2. Now that you have more background information about how your body functions to survive, we'll elaborate on some of the subtle personal indicators of acidosis. The following symptoms of creeping acidosis can be clues that pain and disease may be in your future.

Stiff in the Morning and Loosen Up During the Day
One of the most common acidosis clues is the old
stiff-in-the-morning symptom that we talked about
earlier. Most people aren't too concerned about
moderate morning stiffness — aging and all that. And
most people don't get excited about a weak grip in the
morning. Just a few minutes of activity usually
restores it to full strength. However, flimsy fingers
could well be a precursor to stiff-in-the-morning
which is a precursor to pain and worse. Okay, you
know all that. Now, how does stiffness relate to
acidosis?

Junk!

"Junk" accumulates in your body during the day
as you eat, drink, and nibble at snacks. At night
while you sleep, your body does its housekeeping.
Spent cells and debris from cellular activity are
collected for easy removal when you awaken. That's
the main job of the kidneys.

The kidneys are a "filter system." They remove
substances from the blood that the cells can use and
recycle them through the body to contribute to life
sustaining functions. Materials the body can't use are
eliminated in the urine. However, if the kidneys can't
handle all of the debris that needs to be eliminated
from the body, substances, such as uric acid, are
deposited in the tissue and joints until the night time
housecleaning rush hour is over. So, if the body is
already overly acid and great quantities of dietary
"junk" are present, there's too much "junk" to
prepare for the first exodus in the morning. Some of
it collects in the joints as you sleep. The end result is
morning stiffness.

But internal housekeeping continues while you
are awake. As the day progresses, more and more

"junk" is removed from the body and the muscles and joints "loosen up." Stiffness-in-the-morning each day may be a subtle, short-term inconvenience. However, it is a really big clue that you are eating too much protein.

Most of the "junk" that settles in muscles and joints comes from high-protein foods. Remember, we need protein, but we don't need too much protein. It's debris from too much protein that gives you the rusty-joint feeling in the morning. And if the situation persists, the natural progression moves from stiff-in-the-morning to stiff-and-painful-all-day — every day. Then we call it arthritis.

> **WELLNESS PRINCIPLE:** **Too much protein for too long makes getting up in the morning a pain.**

Urine Smells Like Ammonia

Now we're really getting personal. But this is a BIGGIE! So let's put timidity aside and just launch into this subject. We've gone into this in a couple of places earlier, and now it's time to put it into perspective.

If you were to ask ten people if the odor of ammonia in urine is "normal," very likely at least nine of them would say "yes." And they'd be right, if you consider "normal" to mean the same thing as "usual." However, urine that smells like ammonia may be the norm, but it isn't ever "normal"!

If that's so, why is it so common?

Because most of us eat too much protein and our bodies are struggling to keep our internal acid levels under control.

We talked earlier about the buffering systems that neutralize toxic waste for your internal environmental protection agency. These buffer systems keep your urine pH within a tissue-tolerant range. Strong acid urine (below pH 4.5) will burn delicate kidney tissue. The body doesn't let itself be burned by strong acid if it can help it. So if there aren't enough alkalizing minerals to neutralize the acid left by excess protein foods, a quick, convenient backup system comes to the rescue. The ammonia buffer system.

Cells produce physiological ammonia when they function. This ammonia is handled by the liver. Ammonia can also be produced in the maze of kidney tubules. Physiological ammonia has a pH of about 9.5. That's a strong alkali for the body. When the fluid in the kidneys is too acid, the kidneys produce alkaline ammonia. The ammonia mixes with the acid fluid and the acid is neutralized, or buffered — the pH of the fluid goes up.

The ammonia that neutralizes internal acid is *physiological* ammonia. The body produces it. We're not talking about commercially produced ammonia used as a cleaning agent. Ammonia is ammonia, however, you don't *take* ammonia to neutralize internal acid. It's poison! Granted, ammonia derivatives are used in some medications, but that's not what we're talking about here. The ammonia that neutralizes dietary acid is internally-produced physiological ammonia. Although physiological ammonia is a strong alkali, in the body it combines immediately with acid substances and immediately loses some of its alkaline punch. The point is, you **don't try to put ammonia into your body to neutralize strong internal acid.** When you put acid-producing foods into your body, your body knows how to handle it.

> **WELLNESS PRINCIPLE:** It's up to you to see that your body doesn't have *too much* acid to handle.

Remember, your body is *alkaline by design and acid by function*. Cells produce acid, some foods are acid, and other foods leave an acid ash. Acid produced by cells is eliminated through the lungs. That's no problem. Acid from naturally acid foods, such as lemons, is also eliminated through the lungs. That's no problem either. However, the acid from acid ash foods is in a league by itself. It is neutralized mainly by the bicarbonate buffer system.

The bicarb buffer system has no problem keeping the urine within tolerable pH limits as long as neutralizing minerals are available. However, if too many neutralizing minerals have been used for too long to neutralize the acid of too much dietary protein, the bicarb buffer can't do its job effectively. That's when the ammonia buffer system steps in. The acid neutralized by ammonia is acid from eating too much protein. And, of course, if you don't realize that your diet is contaminating your innards with too much acid, you'll continue to munch away on hamburgers and other high-protein foods. What happens then?

The more protein there is in the kidneys, the more ammonia is produced. This ammonia goes out with the urine. It's a vicious cycle. More protein, more ammonia. In time, ammonia is produced virtually constantly and the urine gives off its tell-tale ammonia odor. So you can see that the odor of ammonia in urine indicates that the body is depending on an emergency backup system to keep dietary acid under control.

The bad news is that this happens in great numbers of people. The worse news is that it can happen in very young children. Diapers that have a strong ammonia odor are a red flag that the child is eating or drinking too much protein. And the worst news of all is that even nursing babies can have ammonia-smelling diapers. This is doubly bad because it means that the mother is eating too much protein and the nursing infant is being affected. Two people are being affected by one person eating too much protein.

The good news is that young children and adults alike can stem the tide of ammonia in the urine. Adding cooked vegetables to the diet is the first step.

WELLNESS PRINCIPLE: **Ammonia odor from the urine is the signal for an immediate change of diet regardless of age!**

WARNING!!   *Ammonia is a poison! It will burn tissue and may be fatal if taken internally! Household ammonia does not neutralize acid in your body!*

Urine That Burns

Burning on urination is generally considered to be a sign of "a bladder infection." The symptom of burning usually responds very well to treatment with appropriate drugs. However, burning urine seems to be a recurring problem. Maybe just making the burning go away isn't the solution. Maybe it isn't a "bacterial" problem after all. Maybe it's a "too much protein" problem and the kidneys are pumping out a steady stream of acid neutralizing ammonia.

Ammonia is a strong alkali. Like strong acid, strong alkali can burn sensitive tissue. But strong alkali is needed to neutralize the strong acid of excess protein. The more acid there is in the kidneys, the more ammonia is produced. So when the body is doing great quantities of ammonia in the urine to keep the kidneys from being damaged, the urine becomes quite alkaline — above pH 8.5. That can hurt and send you scampering to the doctor for relief.

Well, since the body never does anything wrong, why would it dump so much ammonia in the urine that urination is uncomfortable?

To answer a question with a question: Is "uncomfortable" burning urination a threat to the survival of the whole? Probably not. It just hurts. Hurting isn't the body's concern. Survival is. It's much more important to survival for the kidneys to be protected and the urine to be neutralized than it is for the urination process to be comfortable. The body isn't doing anything wrong. It's responding to threatening conditions of the moment.

The solution is simple. Put less acidifying foods and more alkalizing foods into the system and the kidneys won't need to produce great quantities of ammonia to neutralize the acid overload. If great quantities of ammonia aren't produced, there's less ammonia in the urine. When there's less ammonia in the urine, the pH goes down a couple of notches and the burning stops. But it takes a while to relieve burning symptoms by changing your diet. So most people take the short-term "cure" for urine that burns by drinking cranberry juice. That's a faster way to stop the burning. Cranberry juice is great for burning-symptom relief when the burning is due to excess ammonia. However, if the burning continues, consult your doctor.

Cranberry juice is different from orange juice or grapefruit juice and most other fruit juices. Like other fruit juices, cranberry juice is acid going in. However, unlike orange, grapefruit, and most other fruit juices, cranberry juice stays acid throughout the body. The acid of cranberry juice isn't metabolized into carbon dioxide and water the way citric acid is. It goes in acid and stays acid throughout the body. The liquid "acid" that goes in makes a bee-line through the digestive tract. It doesn't go through a long digestion process before it reaches the kidneys. And cranberry juice has only a trace of protein, so it doesn't overexcite the ammonia producing process in the kidneys. It just acidifies the ammonia that's travelling through the urinary tract. Relief!

Drinking cranberry juice to relieve burning urine is a short-term solution to a long-term problem. The problem isn't the highly alkaline ammonia. That's a safe-guard. The problem is the long-term overload of excess protein behind the need for ammonia.

WELLNESS PRINCIPLE: Too much protein can become a burning issue that must be addressed.

Now you can also see why urinary tract infections and burning urine are recurring problems. The symptoms may respond to treatment over and over. However, until the *cause* — excess dietary protein —

is addressed, the symptoms will probably keep coming back.

We've talked about the subtle signs of acidosis that show up as muscle and joint stiffness, urine ammonia odor, and burning urine. Other apparently insignificant signs also pop up frequently. Acid indigestion, "foamy" urine, flatulence. They all come from the same source — acidosis. These private, personal clues are easily ignored indicators that the body is being overstressed. Now you know how your general, overall health can be affected by the internal gyrations your body must go through to handle excess dietary protein. And the best news of all is that you can adjust your intake of dietary protein to allow your body to cruise along more easily without constantly depending on backup systems.

You are now aware of some everyday indicators of acidosis. These indicators are clues that your body is overly acid. An overly acid body must work harder than a slightly alkaline body. This means that the energy that should be available for you to and keep going and going in true Energizer Bunny style is being siphoned off so your internal systems can keep going and going. The food you put into your mouth affects not only how your body works, it affects how *you* work. If your bundle of energy is more like a lump of lethargy, you have a good clue that your body is using much of your energy just to survive your diet.

WELLNESS PRINCIPLE: General fatigue, chronic crashing, or acute weariness indicate an energy drain.

But inappropriate food isn't the sole energy drain for your body. You make food choices every day. You also make choices in the rest of the six essentials. Food and drink are major factors in health, but they don't have the exclusive contract. Health is a whole body condition. Everything you do affects your body. Inappropriate choices in the essentials of exercise, rest, breathing, and thinking can sabotage the effects of the best diet in the world. Your thoughts and attitudes are especially potent health producers or disease directives.

The positive thinking advocates are on the right track. Your thoughts and attitudes have a tremendous impact on the way you live your life and the way you feel about yourself. They also have a tremendous impact on the way your body functions. Constant negative thoughts and attitudes keep your body in a constant state of defense. The internal repercussions of constant defense are ultimately internal exhaustion. That's not a maybe, it's a certainty. And internal exhaustion leads to disease. Adjusting your diet is a lot easier than adjusting your thoughts and attitudes. So thoughts and attitudes take another book.

For now, let's get down to the nitty-gritty of finding out if dietary acid is keeping you and your body from being in top form. On to finding out how the foods you have been eating have affected your body and how you can evaluate your potential for health (pH).

CHAPTER 8

pH — POTENTIAL FOR HEALTH

WHY CHECK URINE pH?

In Chapter 2, you were introduced to the subject of checking your urine to give you an idea of the overall acid-alkaline level of your body. Now the why and how.

Urine is the exit vehicle for much of the debris left from digestion. Everything that enters your body will be used, stored, or eliminated. Urine pH checks focus on the elimination part. Specifically, elimination of the strong acid left after protein has been digested. Most of this acid is processed through the kidneys and eliminated in urine. A small portion is eliminated in the feces. Since most of the acidifying substances from protein digestion are eliminated from the body in the urine, urine pH indicates how well the acid has been neutralized. It also indicates whether the neutralizing was done by minerals of the alkaline reserve or by ammonia. Dietary acid *will* be neutralized. Controlled urine pH checks indicate *how* it's being neutralized in your body.

In the previous chapter we talked about ammonia in the urine. Your cells produce tiny amounts of ammonia in the normal course of business. This ammonia is eliminated. No problem. However, cells don't produce enough ammonia to cause the strong ammonia odor in urine that is generally accepted as normal. The odor comes from ammonia produced in the kidneys as an acid neutralizing backup system. Consequently, a high urine pH number after a controlled urine check indicates that a backup neutralizing process has taken over and your alkaline reserve needs to be replenished. That's the most important piece of information you get from a controlled urine pH check.

WELLNESS PRINCIPLE: Urine pH is the dip-stick for your alkaline reserve.

You have probably noticed the word "controlled" attached to references to urine pH checks. That's because you need to control what goes into your body before you can get an accurate picture of the state of your alkaline reserve. You don't learn anything about the availability of minerals of your alkaline reserve if you check your urine pH just any old time the mood strikes. You need to know what your body has been working on to find out if your alkaline reserve is well supplied. That's the "controlled" part. You control what goes in, and your body responds as best it can. You knowingly "challenge" your body with excess protein that leaves excess acid.

However, before we get too involved in the "how's," here's a very important "Don't!"

If you are very sick, if you have an acute or chronic disease, or if you suspect you have a disease,

DO NOT DO THE URINE pH CHALLENGE!!! That's at least a three-exclamation-point directive. It's not a suggestion; it's a non-negotiable commandment.

If you're sick, your body is already challenged. Your body may not be able to survive the added stress of intentional overacidifying.

If you are sick, you don't need further verification that your body is struggling to survive. You can assume that your internal environment is polluted with too much acid. If you are sick, a concentrated dose of acid ash-producing foods (or strenuous exercise) could push your internal acid level above survival level. Before you even think about taking the urine pH challenge, you must change your diet to begin to refortify your alkaline reserve. Begin by adding one serving of cooked vegetables to your daily diet. That's one (1) serving a day to be added! Not two or three servings or a complete change to only vegetables and fruit. Your body is accustomed to handling the type of foods you eat on a regular basis. Give it a chance to become accustomed to new food. Your body may *need* a quick major diet change, but you won't like the short-term results. You'll be stiff, have headaches or flu-like symptoms, or generally feel worse. So start slowly. After a week, add a second serving of cooked vegetables. Gradually increase the number of servings of cooked vegetables for a couple of weeks. Then add a little fruit.

WELLNESS PRINCIPLE: If you're sick, DO NOT take the urine pH challenge!!!

However, if you are not chronically or seriously ill and are reasonably healthy, take the pH acid challenge to see how well your body is handling your diet.

THE URINE pH CHALLENGE

W hen you get right down to it (whether we want to admit it or not), we take the urine pH challenge test to try to "look into the future." We are really out to reassure ourselves that we are special. We are looking for confirmation that we are healthy, destined for a long, pain-free life, just a tiny bit better than everyone else, and special. Or we are looking for confirmation that we are truly sick, entitled to sympathy, a great deal more burdened than everyone else, and special. However, the pH challenge doesn't predict the future. It is a snapshot of how your body is responding to the types of foods you have eaten in the recent past.

The results of your urine pH challenge may indicate the level of your body's alkaline reserve and its ability to handle acid overload. They don't indicate whether or not you are sick, healthy, or willing to make changes in your diet that will relieve dietary stress. The pH challenge is *not* a diagnostic test. It's an indicator of your alkaline reserve supply — your Alkaline Index™. Helping you to understand what your pH challenge numbers indicate and how you can improve your health is my job. Making the decision to take action on the information is your job.

WELLNESS PRINCIPLE: Information alone won't make you healthy.

The first step of the urine pH challenge is to eat *only* acid ash-producing foods for two full days.

For two days, choose only foods from the list of acid ash-producing foods found at the end of Chapter 3. You are going to deluge your body with "protein-rich" foods. Eat as much of the foods on the acid ash list as you like — meat, pasta, rice, eggs, oatmeal, turkey, bread, or whatever strikes your fancy as long as it's acid ash-producing. But don't eat *anything* listed as an alkaline ash-producing food.

This shouldn't be particularly difficult unless you are a vegetarian. In that case, you may need to make a trip to the grocery store to pluck items from shelves you would ordinarily sail right by.

Suppose you can't bring yourself to do the hamburger, pork, chicken, haddock, or pot roast bit. You can concentrate on grains and nuts — rice, lentils, breads, pasta, cheese pizza, eggs, walnuts, peanut butter, and other high-protein non-meat foods. But no green or yellow vegetables, fruit, or their juice. The acid-producing results of a diet of only grains and nuts are the same as those of a diet of only meats, poultry, fish, and eggs — excess dietary protein and excess dietary acid.

> **WELLNESS PRINCIPLE: Excess protein is excess protein no matter what type of food it comes from.**

What should you drink for these two days? Water, milk, soft drinks, coffee and tea. But no fruit juices!

After two days of intense protein, you're ready for the next step.

Now it's the morning of the third day. Your body's neutralizing capabilities have been thoroughly challenged. Your body has been slaving away surviving a flood of dietary acid. Let's see how the contestants — dietary acid and your alkaline reserve — are doing.

CHECKING URINE pH — THE PROCESS

O n the morning of the third day, your body is saturated with acid from the worst kind of diet. Your urine pH will tell you how it is handling the challenge.

Step 1:   First thing in the morning, after two days of gorging yourself on acid ash foods, you are going to check the pH of your urine when you get up and go to the bathroom.

Step 2:   Have ready for your first voiding: pH test paper in its dispenser, a pencil or pen, and a piece of note paper. The pencil (or pen) and note paper are to record the results. Notice the color chart on the pH paper dispenser. This chart should show color changes numbered in 0.2 increments.

Step 3:   Tear off about a two-inch strip from the roll of pH paper. Holding the strip by one end, direct the other end of the paper into the urine stream very briefly — not more than a second. Just get the pH paper wet. The pH paper does the rest. The color of the paper may or may not change.

Step 4:   Compare the color of the wet pH paper with the colors shown on the pH paper dispenser color chart. Take note of the number above the matching color on the chart. Dispose of the used strip of pH paper. Write on your note paper the date and the number of the color that matched the color from your urine pH test strip.

That's all there is to it.

After you've done the pH test on the morning of the third day, go back to your normal diet. However, after you interpret the results, you may want to change your regular diet to include more body-beneficial types of food. You may not be happy with the results of eating the foods you have in the past. That's why you keep a written record of your challenge results: to see if follow-up tests indicate that your internal environment is improving. As your diet changes, stresses to your body change. Your physiology changes constantly according to the stresses your body is surviving. And your physiology determines your health.

WELLNESS PRINCIPLE: Health is a process.

Now let's look at what controlled urine pH checks indicate.

The pH test paper is specially treated to respond to acidity or alkalinity. When the paper comes in contact with strong acid, it stays yellow. When it comes in contact with strong alkali, the paper turns dark blue. Between the two extremes are variations of yellow through green to blue. The different colors indicate the degree of acidity or alkalinity of the test material, which, in this case, is urine.

While you slept, your body busily gathered internal "trash" from physiological processes and digestion. In the morning, much of the "trash" is eliminated. And since you've poured high-protein food into your body for two days, there's a lot of neutralized acid "trash" to eliminate. The question is: Was the acid neutralized by alkaline reserve minerals or by ammonia? That is the question the color of the pH test paper answers.

Your pH challenge results indicate the availability of neutralizing minerals of your alkaline reserve. We term this availability quotient your Alkaline Index. Your Alkaline Index is an *indicator*. It gives you a general idea of how your alkaline reserve has held up under the diet you've been following.

Your Alkaline Index does not define a specific level of your alkaline reserve. And, **your Alkaline Index does not indicate that you have a disease, much less a specific disease!**

Your Alkaline Index is an *availability indicator*. It *indicates* the amount of alkalizing minerals *available* to neutralize an onslaught of dietary acid. You may have a generous supply of minerals available to neutralize dietary acid. And, then again, you may not. Either way, your body isn't going to let your blood pH drop to critical just because you dumped all that protein into it.

Suppose the neutralizing agents that keep your blood pH under control aren't *available* for buffering protein acid. You still have alkalizing minerals in your bones and other mineral storage bins. But those minerals aren't *available* at a moment's notice to rush in and neutralize the acid from your lunchtime hamburger. It takes a while for the calcium in bones to "change jobs." Your body actually has large stores of alkalizing minerals, but they aren't immediately *available* to neutralize acid. As long as you are alive, you have alkalizing minerals. However, you may not have *available* alkalizing minerals. That's your Alkaline Index — an indicator of your available supply of alkalizing minerals.

FINDING YOUR ALKALINE INDEX

Urine pH challenge numbers fall into three ranges: 5.5 through 5.8, 6.0 through 6.6, and 6.8 and higher. The ranges serve as the basis for your personal Alkaline Index. However, keep in mind that these ranges and your Alkaline Index are significant only after taking the urine pH challenge following two days of eating only acid ash foods. The numbers and ranges are meaningless unless you have thoroughly saturated your body with a concentrated overload of only acid ash-producing foods. You set up the Neutralizing Superbowl. Your survival-oriented body will do whatever it takes to win.

> **WELLNESS PRINCIPLE: Your body works constantly to win the game of life.**

We know that the alkalinity of a substance registers as pH numbers above 7.0. Logic would lead us to conclude that urine pH numbers above 7.0 indicate a healthy alkaline reserve. Through the same logic we might conclude that pH numbers below 7.0 indicate that your alkaline reserve is puny. However, after a major protein challenge to your body, neither

conclusion is correct. The principal concept to keep
in mind when interpreting your urine pH challenge
numbers is that alkaline minerals can neutralize
excess protein acid just enough to keep the acid from
burning delicate tissue. Their neutralizing power is
slight but effective. They can bring the pH of strong
acid up to about pH 6.4, but they can't leap the
neutral pH 7.0 hurdle. As a result, pH challenge
numbers on the acid side of neutral indicate the
strong dietary acid was neutralized by alkalizing
minerals. That's good.

On the other hand, if the alkaline reserve is low
and can't handle the challenge situation, highly
alkaline ammonia does the job. The kidneys produce
a lot of ammonia when excess protein is present.
Ammonia has a pH of about 9.5. Dump significant
amounts of highly alkaline ammonia into an acid
solution and the pH goes up significantly. The result
is urine pH above neutral 7.0. That's not good. We'll
relate that to specific urine pH challenge results later.

> **WELLNESS PRINCIPLE:** **Alkaline minerals neutralize
> slightly; ammonia alkalizes
> dramatically.**

When interpreting urine pH challenge numbers,
there's little difference between pH 6.0 or 6.6. Either
tells the same story. However, if you scored lower
than pH 6.0 or higher than pH 6.6, different stories
are told. When we interpret challenge test numbers,
we are more concerned with a range of pH rather
than with a specific pH number. It's the pH range
that indicates availability of alkalizing minerals.

Since your total alkalizing supply is never
available, we'll say that on an availability scale of 0 to

100, under the best of conditions, only half of the alkaline minerals in your body are available immediately. That would give you an Alkaline Index of 50. So the best results you can get on the urine pH challenge would put you in the pH range of 5.5 to 5.8.

Results of your urine pH challenge in the range of pH 6.0 through 6.6 don't quite reach "good." The pH 6.0 through 6.6 range indicates that your alkaline reserve isn't sufficiently equipped to do the whole job by itself, so ammonia is helping out. That puts you at an Alkaline Index of 25.

The third range of pH challenge results is the least desirable — 6.8 or higher. This shows that ammonia is doing the lion's share of neutralizing. Your supply of immediately available neutralizing minerals is low. Your Alkaline Index is 0. That's not good at all.

So there you have an overview of the relationship between your pH challenge numbers and your Alkaline Index. Now let's look more closely at the meaning of your pH challenge scores and your Alkaline Index.

Urine pH 5.5 - 5.8 — Alkaline Index 50
The best result you can get from the pH challenge is pH 5.5. However, pH 5.8 indicates that your alkaline reserve is holding its own.

If your urine pH challenge scored pH 5.5 or 5.8, your alkaline reserve is adequately available. Your Alkaline Index is 50. You still have enough available alkalizing minerals in your body to handle a concentrated load of dietary acid. Your score shows that you have enough available alkaline minerals to protect your kidneys from being damaged by strong acid from excess protein. Your alkaline reserve is handling acid neutralization without the help of the more potent ammonia backup system.

That's good.

You may have done well on your pH test because you're still young and haven't eaten enough high-protein meals to make major inroads into your alkaline reserve. Maybe you aren't a big meat-eater. Maybe you just like vegetables and fruit. Whatever the reason you fared well, make sure that you continue to re-equip your alkaline supply for the future.

Although your Alkaline Index indicates that your body can handle an occasional glut of protein, you don't need to press the point. If you make a habit of overloading with high protein foods, your supply of neutralizing minerals will slowly dwindle. Your alkaline reserve is adequate — now. Keep it that way. Make sure you eat enough alkaline ash foods to keep it well stocked.

Now that you know your body can handle a sudden burst of excess dietary protein, go back to your regular diet. After a couple of days, check your first voiding urine pH again. But don't expect the same results. Remember, with the pH challenge, your body was processing an overload of protein. On your regular diet, your protein intake should be much less, so your body responds differently. If your follow-up urine pH registers pH 6.2 or lower, you are eating too much acid ash food. You need to reduce the amount of meat, poultry, fish, cheese, and grains and increase the amount of alkaline ash vegetables and fruits. No big deal, just an adjustment in quantities. You don't need to completely stop eating meat or other acid ash-producers. Your body can handle moderate amounts of dietary acid as long as you bolster your alkaline reserve on a daily basis with replacement minerals from vegetables and fruit.

If your regular diet follow-up pH test checks in at above pH 6.2, keep doing what you're doing. You are on the right road. You probably eat generous amounts of vegetables, fruit, and grains, and minimal amounts of meat. If you reduce the amount of grains in your diet, your pH numbers will rise even higher. That's even better.

Keep in mind that these follow-up urine pH numbers from your regular diet apply only if you scored pH 5.5 or 5.8 on the acid challenge test.

Urine pH 6.0 - 6.6 — Alkaline Index 25
Urine pH challenge test results in the range of 6.0 to 6.6 aren't "good." But they're not "horrible." An Alkaline Index of 25 tells you this is the "warning" stage. You started out years ago with a thoroughly competent alkaline reserve. Now, your pH 6.0 to 6.6 shows that your stash of available minerals is dwindling. We might say that the needle on your Alkaline Index "gauge" shows your available reserves are well below "half-a-tank." Although it would *appear* that at pH six-point-something your neutralizing reserve is better equipped than at pH five-point-something, actually, the reverse is true. Your alkaline reserve is running low. However, you still have some alkalizing minerals available.

Very briefly, it works like this: The workhorse mineral of the alkaline reserve — sodium — can weaken strong acid enough to protect your delicate internal tissue. Your alkaline reserve can still neutralize moderate amounts of acid from protein. It can't handle tremendous amounts. But for two days, you filled your digestive system with *excess* protein. There was a lot of rather strong acid — around pH 4.5 — to neutralize. Consequently, if your urine pH is 6.0 or above after eating *a lot* of high protein, something besides alkalizing minerals is working on the acid to bring the numbers up that high. Your alkaline reserve supply either isn't adequate to do the job by itself, or it's just overwhelmed by the volume of acid that needs to be neutralized. So backup systems begin to contribute to the neutralizing (buffering) to get the job done.

If your Alkaline Index is 25, in the past few months you may have noticed some new "signs of aging." You may be stiff in the morning and loosen up as the day goes on. You may tire easily or be short tempered. Your joints and muscles may be painful, you may be more "sickly" than you once were, and you may not sleep as well as you used to. These annoying symptoms are easily passed off as evidence that you're getting on in years. In reality, you are speeding the aging process by eating too much protein. Your alkaline reserves are so low that your body has called on backup systems to help neutralize too much strong dietary acid. Your body is beginning to get tired regardless of your age.

> **WELLNESS PRINCIPLE: Dwindling alkaline reserves can make you feel old no matter how many years you've lived.**

However, your health outlook can be improved rather easily. Reduce the amount of high-protein acid-producing foods and increase the amount of cooked vegetables in your daily diet. Since you probably don't regularly eat many vegetables and fruits, you should gradually reintroduce them to your body. With an Alkaline Index of 25, you'll probably feel better if you eat cooked vegetables rather than raw vegetables and raw fruit. However, that won't always be the case. As your body becomes accustomed to handling more plant food, you'll be able to enjoy a variety of raw vegetables and fruits without suffering "dietary distress of acid indigestion" — that's the politically correct term for "belly ache."

Urine pH 6.8 - 8.0 — Alkaline Index 0

A high urine pH seems to indicate a vast store of alkalizing minerals at work. Not so when you've challenged your body with two days of excess protein. A urine pH score of 6.8 to 8.0 or higher when the body is saturated with dietary acid is very significant. It's the natural downhill slide for your alkaline reserve if your regular diet consists mostly of acid ash foods.

An Alkaline Index of 0 indicates that your *available* alkaline reserve is virtually zilch — gone, depleted, kaput. You may have side-effects that you attribute to heredity, "weak genes," bad luck, or environmental pollution. And, sure enough, environmental pollution is the problem. But it's your internal environment that's polluted. There's more acid "junk" in your internal environment than your diminished alkaline reserve can handle. You may be sick frequently or chronically ill. You may be tired most of the time, have stiff joints, sore muscles, and burning on urination.

**WELLNESS PRINCIPLE: High urine pH after the acid
challenge means a polluted
internal environment.**

A high urine pH following the acid challenge test
of acid ash foods indicates that the important
emergency neutralizing backup system of ammonia is
the principle neutralizer. Instead of minerals
neutralizing the acid from dietary protein, ammonia
is doing the job.

Let's review and summarize:

*After two days of challenging your body with acid
ash foods only,* urine pH can be anywhere from quite
acid (pH 4.5) to slightly alkaline (pH 8.0+). A low
urine pH indicates some alkaline reserve minerals are
still available. But a high urine pH is a warning that:

1. your alkaline reserve is shot and can't
   neutralize the flood of acid sufficiently before
   it gets in the kidneys, or
2. your body is overwhelmed with large
   quantities of protein by-products, so
3. ammonia is produced by the kidneys for last-
   chance acid neutralization.

When ammonia goes out with your urine, your
urine pH numbers are high. And that's why if you
have alkaline urine after eating a lot of high protein
foods, you may have burning on urination. If you
have burning on urination, you may have been eating
too much protein. And it doesn't even need to be
animal protein — just too much protein.

Like the urine of avid meat-eaters, the urine pH
of strict vegetarians can be an ammonia 8.0 with an
Alkaline Index of 0. That's because many vegetarians
are heavy into grains. Their diets revolve around
grains. Grains in all forms. And nuts. Most grains

and nuts are acid ash-producers. Your body doesn't care whether it's fighting too much dietary acid from meat or from grains and nuts. It still goes through the same survival tactics.

Your body is designed to survive. Everything it does is for the sole purpose of survival. And the process of neutralizing acid is a constant. Now you have a method of finding out if your diet is causing your body to depend on emergency backup systems to do one of its day-to-day tasks. You'll find a condensed version of the meaning of your pH challenge results in the Alkaline Index chart on page 144.

WHERE DO YOU GO FROM HERE?

There's not much point in taking the acid challenge unless you do something with the information. You may learn that your diet has been good enough to keep your alkaline reserve well supplied. Or you may learn that your body is losing its constant acid battle.

So, what to do if you "flunked" the urine pH challenge?

Start to improve your diet immediately. But don't toss out all of your acid ash foods and switch cold-turkey to nothing but vegetables. Your body will let you know in a hurry that it isn't accustomed to handling a sudden surge of vegetables and fruits. Your body isn't telling you it "can't" handle a lot of fruits and vegetables. It certainly can. But you probably wouldn't like the short-term results. You see, your body has been working for a long time in its survival mode of constantly coping with excess protein. It's programmed for protein survival. Even if your Alkaline Index is 0 with a urine pH of 6.8 or higher, your body will survive as long as it can. But a quick, radical change in diet can magnify unpleasant symptoms you already have, and add a few that are new. Some of the symptoms that crop up when you change your diet too quickly are rather unpleasant. You'll know you've gone too far, too fast if you develop symptoms such as:

GENERALLY FEELING WORSE   STIFF MUSCLES AND JOINTS
FLU-LIKE MISERIES   BURNING ON URINATION
POUNDING HEADACHES   RAPID WATER LOSS
WHITE COATED TONGUE   CHANGE IN BLADDER HABITS
CHANGE IN BOWEL HABITS   INCREASED IRRITATION
CHANGE IN SEX DRIVE

The objective of diet change is to alkalize your body slowly but surely. Begin immediately, but make diet changes slowly enough to let your body adapt easily. Introduce some of the "more conservative" acid ash foods, such as brown rice, into your diet and add one serving of cooked vegetables to your daily menu for a week. After a week, add another serving of vegetables. Continue the add-a-vegetable-a-week routine for about six weeks. That may sound like a lot of vegetables, but you have three meals a day to work with. Stick with brown rice for a while. You may find the transition to better eating easier with the help of alkalizing nutritional supplements, such as Alka·Line® products designed specifically for that purpose.

Hold off doing another urine pH check for a week or two. Give your body time to adjust. If you re-test your urine too quickly after you start your new eating-for-health program, you may be disappointed if dramatic results don't show up immediately. A gradually improved diet means gradual changes in your urine pH. And the changes at first appear to be backwards. The pattern of change will look as though things are going from bad to worse.

When the out-of-alkaline-reserve bunch improves their diets, urine pH readings go down before they start to come up again. That's because alkalizing minerals are being replenished. As more and more vegetables and fruits contribute precious alkalizing minerals, urine pH goes down, as in the pH 6.0 - 6.6 scenario after the pH challenge. Ammonia isn't the dominant neutralizer. The alkaline minerals are handling some of the neutralizing process. Alkalizing minerals aren't nearly as strong on the alkaline side as is ammonia. So a steady downward trend in urine pH challenge results is great in the short term as you travel the road to health.

Your pH readings should change gradually — one color change at a time. If you are truly committed to improving your diet as a major part of your pursuit of health, you will probably see a dramatic change from your original pH challenge numbers in a couple of months.

A reminder: Your family doctor may not agree with this information, so just try gradually increasing the amount of alkaline ash foods you eat and see how you feel. Remember, your health is your choice. Learn to listen to your body.

WELLNESS PRINCIPLE: Health is not a state of being; it is a state of becoming.

SYNOPSIS OF URINE pH CHALLENGE
1. Eat only acid ash-producing foods for two days.
2. On third day, test urine pH of first morning voiding.
3. Compare color of wet pH paper with color chart on pH paper dispenser to determine pH value of urine.
4. Refer to Urine pH Results chart.
5. Adjust diet according to pH results.

ALKALINE INDEX™ First morning voiding pH Following 2-day Completely Acid Ash Diet			
Alkaline Index	**50** (pH 5.5 - 5.8)	**25** (pH 6.0 - 6.6)	**0** (pH 6.8 - 8.0)
Availability of Alkaline Reserve	Adequate	Limited	Severly Limited
Ammonia	Minimal	Moderate	Maximum
Common Physical Conditions	Occasional aches and pains. Positive attitude. Hyperactive, "Type A" personality.	"Sickly" Frequent joint and muscle pain. Tire easily. Short-tempered.	Frequently ill. Chronic illness. Stiff joints. Sore muscles. Headaches. General fatigue. Usually tired. Urine has ammonia odor. Possible burning on urination.
Recommended Diet Changes	Limit amount of acid ash foods in diet. Increase amount of fruit and cooked veg. Some raw veg are easily tolerated.	Reduce amount of acid ash foods. Increase amount of cooked vegetables. Later, add raw fruit and vegetables.	Immediately reduce amount of acid ash foods. Add cooked veg. Cranberry juice may relieve urinary tract burning.

CHAPTER 9

TIME TO DINE ON ALKALINE

ALKALINITY AND ACIDITY REVISITED

W hy haven't we heard more about this alkaline-acid business? With all of the health tips hurled at us through TV, radio, magazines, newspapers, junk mail, and every other marketing tool available, why don't we hear about the protein paradox or the acid factor?

Economics. The highest acid ash-producing foods (meats, poultry, fish, and grains) are among our biggest money (and influence) producing industries. Try this little experiment: As you watch TV, mentally categorize the food commercials you see as either "acid ash-producing" or "alkaline ash-producing." When not promoting cars, trucks, investment plans, or over-the-counter remedies, the ever-expanding "commercial break" glamorizes major acid producers — fast foods, bigger and better burgers, beef in general, golden fish swished in colorful sauce, and crunchy breakfast cereals adored by children and grown-ups alike. Your informal viewing survey will give you an idea of how much time and money is invested in tilting our national dietary balance to the acid ash side. How many prime-time "commercial messages" sing the praises of fruits and vegetables? Orange juice (a rather substantial industry) and token fruit tossed in with breakfast cereals (another big acid foods industry) occasionally make the big time .

WELLNESS PRINCIPLE: Dollars drive industry, politics, and diet advice.

Most scientists and nutritionists acknowledge the beneficial effects of eating vegetables and the harmful effects of eating meats. If you haven't heard about the connection between meat consumption and heart disease, welcome back from your trip to Mars. But the meat scare doesn't focus on meat itself. First, it was cholesterol. Then triglycerides. Now fat. But cholesterol, triglycerides, and fat are only part of the problem with meat. The biggest problem is the acid-producing protein in the meat itself.

Meat and protein are synonymous. The beef growers can raise leaner cattle to give you leaner meat. And what do you get? Less fat and more protein. That may be helpful in reducing fat intake, but it doesn't help a diet that's top heavy with protein. The only way to get less protein from meat is to eat less meat. And since most of us eat too much protein, most of us should eat much less meat. Is that what the beef industry wants the American public to hear? Not on your alka-life!

Who wants to go up against the great meat industry? Certainly not the government and other powers that be. Politicians can lose dollars if they stray from the meat industry's party line. Researchers can lose grants if they come up with wrong conclusions. So, rather than single out meat as the bad guy in heart disease and other serious illnesses, fats take the rap. We launch on a campaign of counting fat grams. Yet, there's a big difference between hamburger fat and vegetable oil.

Vegetable oils contain no cholesterol. And vegetable oils aren't attached to acid ash-producing animal protein. Of the many vegetable oils on the market, most are better than animal fat, but olive oil is the best. Olive oil has stood the test of time. It has been around at least since Biblical times. Your body needs fats. It just doesn't need too much fat. And it doesn't need animal fat at all.

> **WELLNESS PRINCIPLE: Cholesterol comes in animal products, not vegetable or fruit products.**

Another reason, in addition to economics, you don't hear much about the acid-alkaline question is that it's out of fashion. The concept isn't new. Interest in the body's reaction to alkaline and acid foods has been around for a long time. Now, like the rotary dial telephone, the acid factor is considered a relic of the past. Research into the subject has been shut down for several decades. In the past, research concentrated on the immediate, short-term effects of overloading the body with a lot of alkaline ash or acid ash foods. Investigations dealt with questions having to do with the effect on blood pH of eating large quantities of a particular type of food. But blood pH isn't affected immediately — urine pH is. So the conclusion was that the acid effect of diet is a non-issue. How can this be?

The effect on urine pH of eating alkaline ash foods was discussed in the 1970 book, *Methods in Food Analysis*. The authors noted that a meal of alkaline ash foods affects the urine, but doesn't affect the overall pH of the body. They refer to a 1936 study that "points out that the ingestion of alkali-forming foods in such amounts as a quart of milk, a quart of orange juice, or a pound of bananas does not produce even a temporary shift in the [pH] of the plasma or in the alkali reserve."[2]

This observation contrasted with observations of the effect of introducing sodium bicarbonate and ammonium chloride into the body. (Ammonium chloride is used as an expectorant and as an acidifier.) Forty-five grams of sodium bicarbonate raised blood pH by 0.2, and 15 to 20 grams of ammonium chloride lowered blood pH by the same amount. To drive the point home, the authors write: "To accomplish the same results [0.2 change in blood pH] would require 18 lb of oranges eaten at one time to bring about a shift toward greater alkalinity, and 4 1/2 lb of lean beef or 2 lb of oysters would be necessary to produce an effect comparable to that caused by the ingestion of 15 g of ammonium chloride."[3] Presumably, the quantities "18 lb of oranges" and "4 1/2 lb of lean beef" needed to alter plasma pH were arrived at by extrapolating the alkalizing and acidifying effects of smaller quantities of oranges and beef. It seems unlikely that a researcher's "subject" sat down and ate about 90 oranges or 18 "quarterpounders" to confirm the amounts.

**WELLNESS PRINCIPLE: One meal doesn't change the
pH of the body.**

So, how does all of that "scientific stuff" square
with the concept of eating enough fruits (not 18 lbs at
a sitting) and vegetables to keep your alkaline reserve
well-stocked? Actually, it reinforces what we've been
saying.

First, it confirms that the foods you regularly and
habitually eat affect the pH of your internal
environment — the home neighborhood of your cells.

Second, it demonstrates that adjusting internal
pH through diet is a long-term process. That's the
reason for the recommendation in the previous
chapter that you don't retest your urine pH for a
couple of weeks after taking the urine pH challenge.
Eighteen pounds of oranges might well raise your
internal environment pH by 0.2, but the time needed
to do this would be considerably longer than one
sitting.

Third, reports of yesteryears confirm that your
body responds first to the most urgent needs of the
moment. Take the examples of the sodium
bicarbonate or ammonium chloride that change the
blood pH quickly. They aren't "foods." They don't go
through the same digestion process as solid food.
When you put what we might term "raw chemicals"
into your body, the response is immediate, or at least
faster than the response to foods that go through the
digestion process.

Having said all of that about reinforcing the
concepts in this book, you can see that the concept
of the health implications of acid ash meats and
alkaline ash fruits and vegetables isn't exactly what
some of the "power brokers" of the food industry

want to hear. And what's one of the best ways to discredit financially threatening concepts? Ridicule.

In 1967, Corinne H. Robinson wrote in *Normal and Therapeutic Nutrition*, "Because the body makes [pH] adjustments in the regulation of body neutrality, the reaction of the diet is of no practical significance in health." Then comes the mockery. Robinson goes on to say, "Those who become concerned about the relative acidity or alkalinity of foods have often been misled by false advertising claims of the food quack."[4] Translation: I know best and anyone who doesn't agree with me is a kook with a product to sell.

The book on dietary acid has essentially been closed for the past several decades. But once again, researchers are becoming concerned about the American romance with meat. Murmurs of the relationship between health (especially health care costs) and eating too much meat are beginning to creep into medical circles. If this relationship is openly confirmed in the future, some of us, who for decades have advocated moderation in protein consumption, are apt to lose our "quack" or "nut" status — and I could take that personally. For nearly thirty years I've been labeled by some as "That Nut Who Talks About Eating Too Much Protein." And now, others are arriving at the same conclusion. They may focus on the relationship between protein and specific areas of the body, such as bones, but the connection is being made.

You see, studies such as the 18 pounds of oranges are concerned with one aspect of physiology. And the findings are usually correct — for that one physiological process. But your body's physiological processes are interrelated and survival oriented. The acid factor affects more than just urine or blood pH.

It affects your cells. It affects the workings of *all* of the organs and systems of your body either directly or indirectly. And when your cells, organs, and systems are affected, your life is affected. When your life is affected, your survival potential is affected. And when your survival potential is affected, you begin to notice.

> **WELLNESS PRINCIPLE: We share our body's interest in survival.**

FOOD GETS PERSONAL

Your body is designed to survive. Part of its survival plan is carried out by your very own individual immune system. We might call it the police force of your internal environment. The job of your immune system is to make sure that unwelcome "foreign invaders" are quickly neutralized, subdued, or ousted from your internal community. It happens all the time. Your body is invaded constantly by materials in the air you breathe, on things you touch, and in substances that go into your mouth. It is also invaded when your protective outer layer, your skin, is damaged. Your trusty defense systems are constantly on guard to protect you from the onslaught of potentially dangerous chemical and material riffraff.

Some newcomers to the body are welcome. Minerals and other nutrients from food are potential new members of your body community. But they must be adapted to their new surroundings to be useful, contributing members. They must be personalized before they can benefit your personal internal community of cells. We might say that they become naturalized citizens of your body.

Digestion is more than breaking food down into usable or losable bits and sending them on their way to their proper destination. In the body, food elements must be transformed into individualized material. Fortunately, this happens without you even knowing about it. You just benefit from the results. Food ingredients must be personalized before they are usable.

You see, *you* are a unique individual. You and your body are "in tune" with your own individual world. To become available for your personal use, the elements of the foods, or anything else you put into your body, must adapt to "resonate" with your body. If they don't adapt and get in tune with your personal resonance, out they go. That's why organ transplants are sometimes unsuccessful. The "intruder" is never personalized to be in tune with the surrounding internal neighborhood.

Personalization doesn't happen in a flash. It takes time. That's why you can't expect a quick change in diet to make a quick change in internal pH. A quick diet change will make a quick change in urine pH, but it won't have an immediate effect on the pH of the internal environment. And that's what we're after — improvement in your internal environment to move you toward positive health.

WELLNESS PRINCIPLE: Food elements, like people, must adapt to their surroundings to become part of the community.

APPLIED EATING

It's time to get down to the nitty-gritty of applied eating. You've taken the pH challenge. You've developed a picture of how your body handled more protein in two days than it should have had in a week. And you're either pleased or disappointed with your body's response. But remember: the pH challenge is not a diagnostic procedure. It gives you your Alkaline Index™ — an *indication* of how your body is handling the foods you eat. It doesn't tell you that you are headed straight toward some dread disease or that you are forever healthy and can cancel your insurance.

Whether you scored well or poorly on the pH challenge, it's time to look at some practical ways to help keep dietary stress under control.

We know that vegetables and fruits are the big alkaline ash suppliers. However, most foods, plant and animal foods alike, contain both acidifying and alkalizing substances. And both plant and animal foods provide vitamins and minerals. Much as we champions of fruits and vegetables would like to be able to claim otherwise, plant foods are not the exclusive agents for vitamins and minerals. All foods provide alkalizing and acidifying minerals. However, once they get into the body, most foods tip the scales to one side or the other. For overall health improvement, we're looking for foods that have the best *effect* on your body.

WELLNESS PRINCIPLE: **Your diet goal is to eat foods that tip the scales to the alkaline side.**

The principal alkalizing minerals in foods are sodium, potassium, calcium, magnesium, and iron. We've talked about the neutralizing talents of sodium and calcium. Potassium, magnesium, and iron, while vital to health, aren't as heavily involved in keeping the environment outside your cells slightly alkaline. Potassium, for example, works with the phosphate buffer system inside the cells. But your cells live in the fluid that makes up your internal environment, and your internal environment needs to be slightly alkaline for cells to function effectively. That's where dietary acid is buffered.

The main acidifying minerals in food are phosphorus, chlorine, sulfur, and nitrogen. These minerals appear in the body as phosphates, chlorides, sulfates, and the nitrogen that distinguishes proteins from carbohydrates and fats. Now, lest you forget, protein is good! You need protein in your diet. And you need a variety of proteins from a variety of foods.

Protein comes in many forms to perform many functions in your body. But, since protein has an acidifying effect, you don't need too much protein. High-protein meats have more acidifying sulfur-containing amino acids than do vegetables and fruits. So, we're looking for balance in the *effect* the food you eat has on your body.

ALKADEX VALUES FOR BODY-FRIENDLY MEALS

Wouldn't it be great if there were an easy way to get an idea of the effect food has on your body? Well, there is. It's called the Alkadex™ value of foods. Alkadex values indicate the tendency of foods to alkalize or acidify your body. These values are different from your urine pH or Alkaline Index.

Your Alkaline Index indicates how your alkaline reserve is holding up. But, knowing the level of your alkaline reserve is merely interesting trivia unless you have — and implement — a plan to improve your internal environment. And to plan and implement alkaline eating, you need to have an idea of which foods will have an alkaline effect. The Alkadex values shown in the table at the end of this chapter are the basis for such a plan.

Earlier we talked about most foods having both alkalizing and acidifying properties. Alkadex values indicate the "strength" of the alkalizing or acidifying effect different foods have on your body. Not all alkaline ash foods have the same degree of alkalizing effect. The same holds true for acid ash foods. Some foods have a greater effect than others on either the acid or alkaline side.

The Alkadex value of a particular food gives you an idea of the relative acidifying or alkalizing effect that food has on your body. The Alkadex of a food doesn't indicate grams of protein in that food. And the Alkadex doesn't indicate the pH of the food on your plate. The pH of the food that goes into your body usually has little bearing on the effect that food has on your internal environment. Recall the lemon that is highly acid in its natural state but has an alkalizing effect on the body.

WELLNESS PRINCIPLE: Alkadex values indicate *effects* of food, not grams of protein or pH.

Alkadex values appear as rounded whole numbers. Alkalizing foods have a positive (plus) number. Acidifying foods have a negative (minus) number. It's rather like the numbers in your checkbook. Plus numbers (alkalizing foods) indicate money (minerals) put into your bank (alkaline reserve) account. Minus numbers (acidifying foods) indicate money (minerals) taken out of your bank (alkaline reserve) account. And, like a checking account, ideally, we at least match the ins with the outs to keep the balance from falling below zero.

For example, grilled steak has an *acidifying effect* on your body. The value rating of that effect is an Alkadex of minus twenty-three (-23). To be sure, grilled steak has one of the greatest negative Alkadex ratings even for the meat category — other meats rank more moderately. However, grilled steak is a standard back-yard cookout food and an example of the super-acidifying tendency of many American food favorites. In contrast, broccoli has an *alkalizing effect* Alkadex plus four (+4) on your body.

The greater the plus (+) Alkadex value of a food, the greater the alkalizing effect on your body. The greater the minus (-) Alkadex value of a food, the greater the acidifying effect on your body. The objective is to have at least as great a plus value as minus value overall at each meal. So, if you have that grilled steak at -23 and some broccoli at +4, put them together and you end up with a -19. There weren't enough alkalizing minerals to offset the acidifying elements in the meat. Add a baked potato (+11), lettuce (+8) with salad dressing (-2), and some whole wheat bread (-6), and how does your meal rank on the Alkadex scale? You end up with a -8. The steak, bread, and salad dressing contributed a greater acidifying tendency than the potato and lettuce could offset with their alkalizing tendency. If you consistently run a series of -8 Alkadex meals through your body, before too many years, your alkaline reserve will "yell" for help. You'll hear the "yell" as creaky morning stiffness or other subtle symptom attributed to growing older.

> **WELLNESS PRINCIPLE: The majority of your meals should balance with a "zero" or "plus" Alkadex value.**

"Oh, great!" you think. "Now he wants me to calculate the Alkadex of each meal!"

No, no, no! You don't need to be a fanatical Alkadex counter any more than you need to be a fanatical cholesterol counter, calorie counter, or fat gram counter. Alkadex values are indicators; they aren't to be taken literally. I don't expect you to sit down to your evening meal with calculator in one hand and Alkadex list in the other.

Alkadex values can help you be aware of the tendencies of different foods to affect the alkalinity or acidity of your body. Your meal enjoyment quotient won't suffer at all if you periodically calculate the Alkadex value of your meals for a day or two. That way you can see if the trend of your diet is toward or away from well-balanced alkalinity.

> **WELLNESS PRINCIPLE: Alkadex numbers are clues, not hard evidence.**

Calculating Alkadex values can help you plan meals that will be the most beneficial to you and/or your family. Mothers will find the Alkadex system helpful in preparing alkaline-boosting meals for

children. Children who form a habit of eating
properly may stray from the alkaline path when they
are on their own. But their taste for nutritious food
will have been formed. As Alexander Pope put it,
"Just as the twig is bent, the tree's inclined." With
their tastes "bent" toward alkalizing foods, emerging
adults will be more likely to resume healthful eating
as their "rebellious period" subsides.

Alkadex values can help you to devise more body-
friendly meals than you have probably been eating.
Balance. We're after balance in the foods we eat —
meals that end up with an Alkadex of 0 or higher. For
too long, the typical American diet has clunked the
balance scales heavily toward the acid side. Alkadex
values help you evaluate the potential effect
particular foods can have on the body. They aren't
meant to take the joy out of eating.

Even if you are a vegetarian (hard-core or
moderate), you may be overwhelming your body with
protein. Remember, just about everything you eat has
some protein. Make sure you get *enough* fruits and
vegetables with hefty positive Alkadex values to
counteract the protein's acidifying effects. The old "An
apple a day keeps the doctor away" motto was on the
right track. But, in the long run, one apple a day isn't
going to balance out the effects of eggs, sausage,
pasta, cheese, burgers, and buns. We need to be
aware of the degree of acidifying affect much of the
food we eat has on our bodies and health.

**WELLNESS PRINCIPLE: Alkadex   calculations   are
trend setters.**

EATING AND LIFESTYLE

F ood plays a large part in the lives of most of us. Not only does food taste good, satisfy our hunger, and revitalize us, it is the centerpiece for social occasions. Where do you find the largest knot of people at most social gatherings — around the food table. Informal home parties invariably congeal in the kitchen. Business and social breakfast meetings are part of our social landscape. Lunch hours serve as social interludes in the middle of a work day. Candlelight dinners or fast-food meals are time-honored dating events. Evening TV sessions are the cultural "bring on the snacks" time. We eat, and we eat, and we eat. We use food to grease the wheels of society.

You may have noticed that restaurant meals usually offer little in the way of alkalizing foods. Order a steak dinner and what do you get? Usually a hunk of steak and a few token vegetables just to add color to the presentation of the dish. And since I'm not advocating that you never eat in restaurants, you have your choice of two responses.

(1)   You can eat at only those restaurants that feature a well-stocked veggie menu, or

(2)   You can occasionally enjoy an acid ash meal with all the trimmings and not worry about it.

Worrying about your diet and the amount of acid ash you're getting will cause you more physical problems than the *occasional* high-protein meal. You don't need to eliminate meat completely from your diet. You can eat meat occasionally, as long as you make sure you balance it with plenty of foods from the plant kingdom.

WELLNESS PRINCIPLE: Eating involves more than nourishing the body.

Now that you have been introduced to the acid-alkaline concept, you will look at food differently than you did before. You may have found that the concepts in this book relate to a situation with your own health. Or you may have reservations about the whole concept of alkaline ash and acid ash foods. Either way, you will have a different attitude toward the food you eat every day. The seed is planted. You will at least wonder if the hamburgers, fries, and soft drinks for lunch every day are the ingredients of a potential health time-bomb. You may not eat more vegetables and fruits in the immediate future, but very likely you will at least hesitate over the carrots, broccoli, and dip tray when you're filling your plate at your next party. You may even have a twinge of guilt if you pass up the "live" stuff.

The purpose of this book is not to make you feel guilty about eating "wrong" types of foods. In the long-run, guilt feelings are more powerful "acidifiers" than acid ash foods. So no matter what foods you choose to eat, eat them, enjoy them, and when you're finished, toss the guilt into the trash with the other garbage. The purpose here is to help you understand that the types of food you eat make a big difference in how your body functions.

There's more to life than eating. You don't need to be a fanatic about eating only alkaline ash foods. Indulge yourself occasionally and enjoy it. And you don't need to alienate family and friends by harping on the perils of their bad diets, or sermonizing on the virtues of veg.

Eating is just one facet of lifestyle. While it is very important — principally because we do so much of it — eating only good, nourishing, alkaline ash-producing, foods will not assure you of outstanding health, happiness, and success, or winning the lottery. Your life includes choices in the rest of the six essentials. No matter how well you eat, if you abuse your body by not giving it opportunities for adequate rest and exercise, or if you subject your lungs to constant pollution, you reduce the positive effect of the good food. And, most important, you can't eat enough good food to neutralize the disastrous health effects of constant "acid thinking." Guilt, fear, worry, anxiety, hate, jealousy, hopelessness, and low self-esteem are just a few examples of "acid thinking." These negative emotions can escalate into negative attitudes.

Negative attitudes can become the filter through which all thoughts and observations pass. Negativity becomes a habit. And negative thoughts and attitudes excite strong physiological responses of defense. So, if all day, every day, you find fault with yourself and others, you keep your body in constant defense. It's ready to do battle or run. But you're a civilized creature. So your body doesn't do either. Defensive energy is generated with no place to go. And you wonder why you are nervous, up-tight, tired, and plagued by "indigestion," high blood pressure, meandering aches and pains, or the blahs. An apple a day, or 18 pounds of oranges, won't protect your body from the effects of constant physiological defense.

WELLNESS PRINCIPLE: **The best diet in the world can't rein in galloping negativity.**

Does that mean that if your family life, job, or the general world situation keeps you up-tight and stressed there's no point in trying to upgrade your diet?

Not at all. Stress is a fact of life. Your body is designed to handle stress. However, if you improve your diet but you don't notice an improvement in your health or your Alkaline Index, your thoughts and attitudes are probably the *cause* of your problem.

That doesn't mean you should go back to an acid ash-based diet. Why inflict dietary stress along with mental stress on your one and only body. It needs to last you a lifetime.

Fortunately, you are in charge of your health. You have freedom of choice as far as what you eat, drink, and think. You also have freedom of choice in how you exercise, rest, and breathe. You can choose to smoke or not smoke cigarettes. You can choose to live or work in an overly polluted area. You don't need to depend on others to make these choices for you, so you don't have to live with the consequences of the decisions of others.

With freedom comes personal responsibility. If you aren't feeling as good as you would like, if you don't have as much energy as you would like, it's up to you to do something about it. The types of food you are eating may be the major problem. Diet is relatively easy to change. It's a good place to start. Now that you have a nodding acquaintance with the acid factor in foods, you can improve your diet to improve your body's internal environment. And if you are really intent on giving your body the best of everything in life, you can improve your outlook — your view of your external environment. But we'll leave that subject for another book.

Now, let's see about devising a game plan to help you make the transition to eating the types of foods that will help your internal environment. Who knows, once you make the change and feel better, your outlook may change, too.

ALKADEX™ OF SELECTED COMMON FOODS

Positive Alkadex Foods*
Alkalizing Effect on the Body —
Plus (+) Values

Apples	+3	Cider, apple	+4
Artichokes, boiled	+8	Cola beverage	+3
Avocado	+11	Coconut	+5
Bamboo Shoots	+7	Shredded	+4
Bananas	+6	Dried	+9
Beans, baked	+3	Milk	+8
Butter, boiled	+6	Coffee, beverage	0
Lima, fresh	+14	Cucumbers, fresh	+4
Kidney, canned	+3	Dates	+11
Navy, canned	+3	Eggplant	+5
Snap, raw	+5	Figs, dried	+36
String	+5	Fruit salad, canned	+3
Broccoli	+4	Gingerbread	+9
Brussels Sprouts, boiled	+1	Grapes, Black	+7
Cabbage	+6	White	+6
Spring, boiled	+1	Grapefruit	+6
Winter, boiled	+5	Grape-nuts®	+1
Red	+4	Guava	+7
Cantaloupe	+8	Honey, Dark	+2
Carrots	+10	Light	+1
Young, boiled	+6	Horseradish	+4
Cauliflower	+3	Kale	+13
Boiled	+2	Kohlrabi	+6
Celery, raw	+8	Leeks	+6
Boiled	+5	Lemons	+8
Leaves and stalks	+3	Lemon juice	+4
Cherries, Black	+3	Lentils, boiled	+1
Sweet	+5	Lettuce	+8
Chestnuts	+9	Orange Marmalade	+3

Milk	+2	Chips	+19
Molasses	+49	Pumpkin	+3
Mushrooms	+4	Radishes, red	+7
Muskmelon	+8	Raisins	+25
Nectarines	+6	Raspberries	+6
Okra	+5	Rice pudding	+2
Onions	+1	Romain	+7
Oranges	+6	Rutabagas	+9
Orange Juice	+5	Sauerkraut	+6
Parsnips	+7	Spinach	+15
Passion Fruit	+9	Boiled	+40
Peaches	+6	Squash, Hubbard	+3
Canned	+4	Strawberries	+3
Pears	+3	Tangerines	+6
Peas, fresh	+1	Tomato	+6
Pineapple, fresh	+6	Turnips, boiled	+5
Canned	+2	Vinegar	+1
Potatoes, Sweet, baked	+8	Watercress	+8
White, baked	+11	Watermelon	+2
Boiled, new	+7		

Negative Alkadex Foods*
Acidifying Effect on the Body —
Minus (-) Values

Anchovies, salted	-13	Beer	-1
Bacon, cooked	-10	Biscuit, baking powder	-4
Barley, boiled	-6	Bologna	-9
Beef, corned	-14	Bread, white	-2
Roast, med. fat	-21	Bread, whole wheat	-6
Roast, fat	-12	Cake, chocolate	-3
Misc. fat free cuts	-12	Sponge	-11
Porterhouse	-11	Carp	-20
Ribs, med. fat	-14	Caviar	-12
Round steak	-11	Cheese, Cheddar	-5
Steak, grilled	-23	Stilton	-8

Chicken, roast	-25	Margarine	-1
Cod, fried	-16	Mayonnaise	-1
Grilled	-22	Mushrooms, fried	-2
Corn, sweet	-2	Mustard	-31
Crab, boiled	-40	Oatmeal	-2
Crackers, Graham	-9	Oysters	-14
Saltines	-8	Pancakes	-2
Cream of Wheat®	-10	Peanut butter	-4
Doughnuts	-2	Peanuts	-12
Duck, roast	-24	Pork	
Egg, whole, boiled	-16	Chops, grilled, lean	-13
Fried	-17	Loin, roast	-15
Poached	-20	Sausage, fried	-4
Scrambled	-13	Rice, white, boiled	-8
White	-5	Salmon, steamed	-16
Yolk	-33	Canned	-20
Eggnog	-10	Sardines, canned	-27
Farina, cooked	-2	Scallops, steamed	-36
Filberts	-2	Semolina	-7
Flounder, steamed	-20	Shredded wheat	-6
Fried	-14	Shrimp, cooked	-2
Flour, Graham	-11	Sole	-16
White	-7	Sorghum	-1
Whole wheat	-3	Spaghetti, cooked	-2
Haddock	-15	Toast, white	-2
Halibut, steamed	-19	Whole wheat	-7
Ham, smoked, med fat	-8	Trout, sea, steamed	-22
Hazelnuts	-4	Turkey	-18
Hot dogs	-10	Veal	-13
Lamb	-10	Venison, roast	-24
Liver, calves, fried	-50	Waffles	-6
Lobster, boiled	-38	Walnuts, English	-8
Macaroni, cooked	-1		

*Alkadex™ values are estimated indicators of the relative alkalizing or acidifying effect particular foods have on the body. They are not intended as definitive measurements of the nutritional value of foods.

Alkadex values are intended to provide a basis for evaluating the relative alkalizing or acidifying effect on your body of the foods you eat. They are general indicators. They are not intended to be used for mathematical calculations to reach a positive value for each meal.

CHAPTER 10

AN APPLE A DAY?

GAME PLAN FOR HEALTH

An apple a day is an asset to your diet. But one, lone apple paddling in a sea of acid ash producing foods can't overcome alkaline reserve abuse. You need more alkaline ash food than that. However, you don't need to constantly grapple with grams to construct healthful, satisfying meals. Menus needn't be planned down to the last Alkadex number. Body friendly eating evolves easily when you are aware of the alkalizing or acidifying tendencies of foods, keep the 70-30% rule in mind, and make more alkaline reserve deposits than withdrawals. Meal planning shouldn't be a burden. A little flexibility goes a long way. Eating is both a necessity and a recreational sport.

WELLNESS PRINCIPLE: **Your diet should follow a game plan, not a battle plan.**

Now that you have had an opportunity to look over the Alkadex values of various foods, you may have noticed some values that don't seem "just right." Chicken, for instance. Roast chicken has a greater negative value than roast beef. How can that be? We are being told by the "health experts" to eat more chicken and less beef.

That's the key. "Health experts" these days focus on fat consumption. Alkadex values are based on comparable quantities of the foods listed, and pound for pound, chicken has less fat than beef. But, how often do you order a 10-ounce slab of chicken? We often eat less chicken at a meal than we do beef. However, since chicken has less fat, chicken has a greater acidifying tendency than beef. But that doesn't mean you shouldn't eat chicken. It means that you shouldn't eat too much chicken, and you should balance the chicken you do eat with foods with positive Alkadex values.

While we're on the subject of fat, look at the positive Alkadex value of potato chips. Wow! It's +19. That would seem to indicate that we can crunch potato chips all day long and really fortify our alkaline reserves. And that's partially right.

Indeed, potato chips rank high on the Alkadex scale, but they also rank high in fat and sodium. Your body doesn't need the concentrated amounts of fat and sodium that give potato chips their taste appeal.

Another question-raising food on the positive Alkadex list is spinach. The positive Alkadex value of "Boiled" spinach is nearly three times that of "Spinach." Sounds strange until you realize that raw spinach "cooks down." You can have a plateful of raw spinach, but when that amount is cooked, you end up with a few spoonsful, or forksful as the case may be. So the higher Alkadex value for cooked spinach is a function of volume.

And again, just because boiled spinach shows a high Alkadex value, that doesn't mean it's the best food for you. Spinach contains oxalic acid which can leach calcium from your body. So when you eat spinach, reinforce your calcium supply with foods such as beans.

You can see by these examples of chicken, potato chips, and spinach that Alkadex values are best used to indicate trends. Not as the sole criterion for food selection.

WELLNESS PRINCIPLE: **Alkadex values are guides, not dictators.**

The menus in the following chapter — Starter, Regular, and Maintenance Menus — are the fundamentals of your alkalizing game plan.

The first step of any plan is to determine the end result you want to achieve. The overall objective of your eating plan is to alkalize your body. Your individual objective and how you go about reaching it depend upon how you fared with the pH challenge.

If your Alkaline Index was 50, your objective is to keep it that way. Your alkaline reserve is still in good shape. Is it in good shape because you eat a lot of alkaline ash foods? Or is it in good shape now because you eat some alkaline ash foods and are young enough that the decline in the net worth of your alkaline reserve hasn't yet become apparent? Either way, begin with the Starter Menus to help your body adjust easily to a regimen of alkalinity. After several days, move on to the Regular Menus and, later to the Maintenance Menus as meal guides to help keep your alkaline reserve solvent.

If your Alkaline Index was 0 or 25, your objective is to begin immediately to rebuild your alkaline reserve. The first step is to recondition your body to handle more alkaline ash foods. The Starter Menus will help to get you eating in the right direction. After a week or so, as you — and your body — become accustomed to your new way of eating, advance to the Regular and Maintenance Menus.

WELLNESS PRINCIPLE: **Replenish your alkaline reserve by refurbishing your menus.**

CHOICE EATING

We have said that eating is one of the six essential areas of life. You make eating choices constantly. So you might as well make choices of foods that will help your body work better, help you feel better, and help you enjoy your stay on this planet. In other words, you may as well design your meals around an effective alkalizing diet program.

For most people, the word "diet" has a negative connotation. It's a word generally associated with restrictions and the rule "If you like it, you shouldn't eat it." However, the alkalizing eating program described here is not intended to be an exercise in self-denial. It is intended to be a reconditioning program. Most people who follow this alkalizing program find that before long, their eating isn't "restricted" at all. As their bodies become accustomed to processing more alkaline ash foods than in the past, their appetite for acid ash foods usually dwindles.

WELLNESS PRINCIPLE: **Your body adapts to processing the types of foods you regularly give it.**

The alkalizing program described here is designed to "reprogram" your body's inherent processing skills. Instead of processing mostly acid ash foods, your body is "retuned" to process mostly alkaline ash foods. But a word of caution. There may be a conversion period. The first few days you may not feel as good as you did before you began the program. However, the conversion period usually lasts no more than a few days. It's smooth sailing after that. So if you feel sluggish or generally "blah" soon after you begin your alkalizing program, that's good. It's a signal that your body is ridding itself of toxic materials and reactivating your body's ability to use the enzymes required to process more appropriate types of food. It's a signal that you really needed to make different food choices.

This eating program serves as a tune-up for your body. It is a thirty- to sixty-day alkalizing, energizing, weight control program. If you follow this program for thirty to sixty days, you will probably notice a change in your weight as well as your energy level. Your energy level should rise. And if you are overweight, don't get excited if you gain a couple of pounds in the beginning. In the long run, you'll probably lose some excess pounds. The menus of this eating program provide for daily calorie intake between 1250 and 1500. And since only a small amount of animal protein is included, few of the calories are from fat. My experience has shown that slightly alkaline bodies are less likely than acidic bodies to retain fat.

If you're underweight, you, too, may gain a few pounds. Although the calorie level is relatively low, the nutrition-availability level is high. Your body will "soak up" nutrients your cells need and you may add a few pounds.

WELLNESS PRINCIPLE: **A slightly alkaline body seeks its optimum weight.**

I have stressed the need for a well-balanced diet. Your body needs dietary fat, protein, and carbohydrates. The 1250 to 1500 daily intake of calories in this program offers that balance. Daily menus are geared to provide about 10 grams of fat, 30 grams of protein, and 250 grams of carbohydrate. These quantities fall into general guidelines for healthful, energy building, weight control eating. If your lifestyle includes strenuous physical activity, you may need to adapt your calorie intake to suit your individual needs. Marathon runners, farm workers, professional dancers, and other "busy bodies" are inclined to burn more daily calories than non-exercising "desk jockeys."

One of the main objectives of this body tune-up plan is to alkalize your body. To help jump-start your tune-up, the daily menus call for substituting one or two meals a day with an alkalizing meal replacement, such as Alka·Slim™. An alkalizing meal replacement in your daily diet helps balance negative Alkadex foods you might include in the day's "solid food" meal.

For busy days when you can't fit the alkalizing meal replacement into activities such as a civic club breakfast, business lunch, and dinner with guests, all is not lost. When you make your food selections, be sure you eat more foods shown on the Alkaline Ash-Producing and Positive Alkadex lists than on the Acid Ash-Producing and Negative Alkadex lists.

WELLNESS PRINCIPLE:　　**A variety of alkaline replenishing foods means a variety of nutrients.**

The sample menus shown in the next chapter are designed to accomplish three goals.

First, to show that you can eat flavorful, satisfying meals while restocking your alkaline reserve. You may be surprised to find the occasional meat product sprinkled in with the plant food. Total abstinence from meat is not necessarily the solution to all of life's ills and miseries.

Second, to give you a jumping off place for designing your own alkaline ash-based meals. The majority of people in this country usually answer the question "What's for dinner?" with the name of a meat, poultry, or fish dish. These alkalizing menus can help you begin to reprogram your thinking by shining the dinnertime limelight on assorted vegetables.

And, third, to reinforce the concept that you don't need to count ounces, grams, calories, or Alkadex values for the rest of your life to plan healthful meals. Variety in alkaline ash-based meals gives you needed nutrients and amino acids without overloading on fat, cholesterol, sodium, or calories. And as long as you don't overeat, your weight is more likely to find its

appropriate level when you get most of your nutrition
from low-calorie, cholesterol-free plants.

Nationally, the focus of planning healthful menus
is changing from meat-based meals to vegetable-
based meals. Yet, the need for a well-balanced diet
hasn't changed. In your zeal to follow a healthful diet,
make sure you include fat, carbohydrate, and protein
— but not too much of any of them. Too much fat —
especially animal fat — will clog your arteries. Too
much carbohydrate will add pounds. Too much
protein will acidify your body.

WELLNESS PRINCIPLE: **℞ for healthy eating:
moderation and balance.**

Remember, the eating program described in the
next chapter is a short-term program — thirty to
sixty days. For most people, that's how long it takes
to begin to reinforce their alkaline reserves and
become quite comfortable with their new way of
eating. After your break-in period of thirty to sixty
days, you'll be designing your own menus. That's a
good time to calculate the approximate Alkadex value
of your meals for a day or two. It will tell you if the
trend of your diet pattern continues to lean toward
the alkaline side. But there's no need to make
Alkadex calculations a habit. The Alkadex list is
intentionally limited. It shows only some of the foods
common to American meals. Some of the foods listed
may be regional rather than national favorites. This
limited list can help you to arrive at a "ballpark"
Alkadex value of your regular meals. That's what
you're after — trends, not "actual" Alkadex values.
The question you want to answer with Alkadex values

is "Does my diet *tend* to replenish, or reduce, my alkaline reserve?"

You and your family are more likely to form habits of alkaline eating when you devise meals that suit your tastes. Create meals that are appealing, tasty and satisfying. Here are some tips to add flavor to your alkalizing program.

- Steaming is the preferred method of preparing vegetables.
- Most vegetables have little aroma until they are cooked.
- Most fresh vegetables have a gentle flavor if not overcooked.
- To keep from overcooking fresh vegetables, remove them from the heat when you can smell them.
- Spices and herbs add flavor to food.
- Use only enough spices and herbs to enhance — not overpower — the flavor of your food.
- Most spices and herbs are not protein, fat, or carbohydrate intensive, and have fewer negative side effects than salt which promotes fluid retention.
- Spices that add a hint of sweetness to food include allspice, cinnamon, ginger, mint, nutmeg, clove, and cardamom.
- Celery, parsley, or fresh lemon juice can give foods a salty flavor.
- Hot spices, such as chili, red pepper, or cayenne can satisfy a craving for salt.

CREATIVE EATING

Most of us won't follow through with a revised eating plan unless it is pleasant, satisfying, and obviously beneficial — or we are threatened with dire consequences. For example, a sixtyish man has a tendency to listen and swear-off meat when told by a doctor to cut down on fat consumption or risk a heart attack in the near future. A severe diabetic has little trouble eating foods that help keep his blood sugar under control. But, we're not talking here about trying to "treat" a disease by diet. We're talking about feeding your body the most beneficial types of foods *before* symptoms appear. To stick with the new regime, it must be pleasant and satisfying.

WELLNESS PRINCIPLE: **A remedial diet is easier to follow when the threat to survival is obvious.**

If you have been one of the "It's not a meal without meat" set, you may not be excited about converting to meatless meals on a regular basis. But, again, if you wean your body off meat slowly, before long you will find that you want less and less meat. And, again, if you are now "reasonably healthy," you don't need to be completely "meat-free" for the rest of your life.

In contrast to the "I can't give up my meat" mindset is the exuberant "vegetarian convert." Some people become so enthusiastic about trying to "eat healthy" that they decide to eat nothing but vegetables and fruits — no meats, no grains, no nuts. If you take this route, your appetite probably won't be satisfied, and you will deny your body some of the nutrients it needs. You need balance in your diet. Every day, you lose protein from your body. This protein needs to be replaced — but not ten-fold. You need protein and other nutrients from grains. Be sure you include grains and nuts with your alkalizing vegetables and fruits.

Once you begin to look at foods as alkalizers or acidifiers and make food choices accordingly, you will find that you gravitate toward the alkalizers. One of these days, you will realize that you are programming your meals and snacks to the alkaline side without thinking about it. "Good" food selection becomes automatic. And you will find that when you do eat an acid ash meal, you don't feel quite as good as usual.

WELLNESS PRINCIPLE: **A body accustomed to "good" food lets you know when you've strayed too far.**

DESIGNATED DRINKING

What's the best liquid refreshment to go along with your new eating plan?

You guessed it, water.

Water accounts for just over half of your body weight — 57% according to one source. The chemical reactions in your body take place in a water medium. So you need water. Clean, pure water.

But there's a problem here. On the way to our advanced technological society, we managed to thoroughly abuse our planet's water supply. Completely pure water is a thing of the past. Even the

snow on the highest mountain top isn't as pure as it
once was. However, generic man is ever up to a
challenge. Technology has abused our water supply,
and technology has devised ways to minimize the
effects of that abuse.

WELLNESS PRINCIPLE: **Technology gives, and
technology takes away.**

In our country, the water most of us drink is
treated to nullify the effects of the micro-critters that
can create havoc in our bodies. Chlorinated water
flows freely from the taps in cities throughout the
country. So that's what most of us drink. Indeed, in
technologically advanced countries such as ours,
chemical water treatment has virtually eliminated the
devastating health problems that come from drinking
polluted water. And in this case, the cure is not
worse than the disease. Drinking chlorinated water is
better than drinking water contaminated with raw
sewage and other pollutants. But the cure for water
pollution isn't complete. Researchers have found a
relationship, in chickens, between chlorinated water
consumption and depression of High Density
Lipoproteins — HDLs, the "good" cholesterol that
"protects" against coronary heart disease. Granted,
we aren't chickens. But the effects were on the
cholesterol, and we have that. Chlorinated water is
not the best liquid to pour into your body day after
day, year after year.

So what do you drink?

Fruits and vegetables.

"Do you mean fruit and vegetable juices?" you
ask.

Yes, you can do that. However, when your diet is fruit and vegetable based, you get water with your food. Fruits and vegetables come with built-in water. And it's the best kind. The water in fruits and vegetables has been filtered through the plant. It is pure. And there's a good bit of it. So when you switch to an alkaline ash diet with plenty of fruits and vegetables, you reduce the amount of liquid you must add separately.

Most of us have heard or read that we should drink eight glasses of water a day. Not a bad idea — if you eat the kinds of foods most Americans eat. But when you eat mostly plant food, you need to drink only when you're thirsty. And you won't be nearly as thirsty as you were when your diet was meat, poultry, and fish based.

To illustrate the difference in "drinkability" of foods, your lunchtime hamburger patty is 54% water. White bread is 37% water. Compare that with the 71% water in a baked potato with skin, and 84% water in an apple. You can see why you don't get as thirsty when you eat vegetables.

WELLNESS PRINCIPLE: An apple a day is a nutritious, thirst-quenching "drink."

As a practical matter, however, we do get thirsty. So what's the best kind of water?

Reverse osmosis — RO — water. RO water is another technological innovation. Water is filtered through a special membrane that removes the substances you don't need in your body. And it "cleans" the water without "killing" it. RO water

purifiers are available for home use. (Some RO
sources are shown in the Appendix.)

Distilled water has long been a favorite of the
health-conscious. However, distilled water is "dead."
In the distillation process, the "life" goes with
everything else. That's why distilled water tastes
"flat." It is "flat." You can revitalize distilled water by
adding fresh lemon juice. Revitalized distilled water is
second best to RO water.

Your body doesn't need coffee, tea, or soft drinks.
Decaffeinated or not, they stimulate your body
unnecessarily. And most soft drinks contain
phosphoric acid. Another acid your body doesn't need
to contend with. However, coffee, tea, and soft drinks
are fixtures of modern-day America. None of them
will make you healthier. But in very moderate
quantities, they probably won't do you serious harm.
The crucial phrase there is: "in very moderate
quantities." Your body is designed to survive these
indiscretions, but don't get carried away.

And then there's milk. If you're over two years
old, your body doesn't need milk. Earlier, we talked
about the acidifying effects of cow's milk. Milk is a
full-time resident of most American refrigerators.
Nevertheless, in my opinion, milk should not be
consumed by adults. Nor should it be a staple for
children once they begin to get teeth. The short-term
effect of drinking cow's milk may be slight alkalinity.
However, the long-term effect of all that protein in
cow's milk puts an unnecessary stress on the body's
buffering systems. And that's doesn't take into
account the effects of pasteurization.

Cow's milk is not good food for humans.
Pasteurized cow's milk isn't good food for calves.
Calves that have been fed pasteurized milk can

survive for about six months. That's it. Calves can't survive on pasteurized cow's milk. Pasteurization affects the way the minerals in the milk are held together. Calcium in pasteurized cow's milk may not be as usable as it was before the milk was "cooked." So, that milk sitting in your refrigerator isn't the wonder food you have been led to believe. It may not kill you, but in the long run, it may not do you as much good as you thought.

WELLNESS PRINCIPLE: **As a health food, milk is the Great White Hoax.**

And what would a section on "drinking" be without a word about alcoholic beverages? The reaction of alcohol in the body is similar to that of the reaction of white sugar. It is pure energy. It goes in and is converted immediately to energy. This conversion to energy process requires minerals, vitamins, and enzymes, none of which is supplied by the alcohol. Alcohol is a "negative" energy substance. You get a temporary spurt of energy, but your body loses more than it gains. Alcohol stimulation is usually followed by a let-down.

However, if you enjoy a glass of wine or social drink occasionally, I am not advocating complete abstention. You don't need to rigidly resolve to never take another alcoholic drink. You can, but that won't guarantee good health any more than rigidly resolving to never eat meat again. Moderation is the byword. If you deny yourself every small pleasure in a crusade for health, you're not living — you're existing.

Health is a function of balance. I can't think of anything that isn't illegal or immoral that I would advocate giving up completely — except smoking cigarettes. Moderation is the key. Treat yourself occasionally to the food and drink you enjoy but have chosen not to eat regularly. And when you treat yourself, enjoy it! Then get back to body-friendly eating and drinking, enjoy it, and let your body survive in comfort. You'll know when you're doing right.

> **WELLNESS PRINCIPLE:** **Eat when you're hungry; drink when you're thirsty; listen to your body.**

THE RESPONSIBILITY SHIFT

So there you have it. The meat and potatoes of healthful eating. Too much meat and not enough potatoes and other veg can lead you down the garden path to an acid existence. You choose the substances your body must process. Choose lots of vegetables and fruits and your body gets the minerals and other nutrients it needs to survive easily and reasonably well. Burden it with too much protein and your body will survive, but eventually organs, systems — and you — will become exhausted. You are responsible for your health. But you don't need to carry around an instruction book to build health. Once you've grasped the two basic concepts of healthy eating, you can adapt your diet to your individual tastes. And those basic concepts are: Your body is *alkaline by design and acid by function,* and your body is designed to survive. Survival of the acid generated by physiological function and the acid of most naturally acid foods is a breeze. It's exhaled. The acid left by acid ash foods drains your alkaline reserve. Simple as all that.

Having said all that, keep in mind that although diet is very important, it is not the answer to all physical ills. Even the best diet can't undo the crippling effects of accidents, injuries, birth defects, and other major damage. However, a diet that's low in nutritional stress can help even a damaged body to reach its greatest potential.

WELLNESS PRINCIPLE: **You have your own individual potential for health.**

Your body's survival responses are perfect for every stimulus it receives. This book focuses on food and drink stimuli. But your body receives stimuli from many other sources, including the rest of the six essentials. It's up to you to make sure it is fed the best stimuli possible. It's up to you to see that you give your body proper rest and exercise, and clean air. And even more important, it's up to you to feed your body health-producing mental stimuli. Positive thoughts are low-stress thoughts!

The mental conversations you have with yourself have a greater affect on your health than the food you eat. So if you took the pH challenge, now eat mostly alkaline ash foods, have improved your urine pH numbers, but still don't feel as well as you would like, you may be experiencing emotional override. Physiological responses to your thoughts and emotions are overriding the beneficial effects of the alkaline reserve-replenishing diet. Physiological survival responses are automatic. You have virtually no conscious control over internal survival processes.

You can control many of the stimuli your body must survive. Diet stimuli are among the most easily controlled. However, emotional override can keep you from feeling your best even when you eat the most body-friendly diet in the world. You can't reach your greatest potential for health while emotional override dominates your physiology. But that doesn't mean you should scrap your healthy eating program. Going back to an acid ash diet will just make the situation worse.

WELLNESS PRINCIPLE: **Emotional override coated with an acid ash diet makes a potent pain producer.**

Emotional override isn't a "mental disorder." The common term for emotional override is "stress." We're not talking about "mental illness." That's an entirely different situation. Mental illness and/or brain disorders require the help of competent specialized professional help. The focus here is on how the stress in your life affects your overall health.

Explaining why and how thoughts, feelings, and emotions affect your overall health requires a book in itself. The whole-body effects of stress-induced emotional override are the subject of my book *Dynamic Health: Using Your Own Beliefs, Thoughts and Memory to Create a Healthy Body* (1995). For now, we'll just say that thoughts, emotions, and attitudes wreak more havoc on your body and your pH than any of the other stimuli your body receives. If your aches, pains, and zero energy level are the consequences of emotional override, take heart. You

are not alone. If my clinical experience is any
indication, most people living fast-paced, stress-filled
lives are trying to deal with emotional override
whether they realize it or not. And even those whose
lives are less frantic — on the surface — may be
plagued daily with symptoms of emotional override.

You can determine if your emotions are
overriding the beneficial effects of your diet by a
simple saliva pH test. The details of this test are
explained in my *Handbook for Monitoring pH, Your
Potential for Health* (1996). Again, this is not a test to
replace the services of a professional mental health
specialist. It is a test to evaluate whether diet or
emotions dominate your physiology.

Food, drink, and thoughts are the most potent of
life's stress generators, but they are only three of the
six essentials of life. Health — or disease — is a
whole-body condition. Everything you do, think, and
eat affects your physiology and your body. You need
a well-rounded diet *and* a well-rounded life.

The concepts outlined in this book can help you
to revamp your eating habits to make your diet as
body-friendly as possible. As long as you are going to
eat anyway, you may as well give your body the types
of foods it can use best. You can't eliminate stress
from your life, or your body. But you can reduce the
amount of nutritional stress your body must survive.

You have only one life on this planet (that we
know of). You may as well live it as comfortably and
productively as possible. If you are beginning to
notice subtle symptoms that your body is
overstressed, it's time to do something different in
your life. When you make inappropriate choices, you
can't continue to do everything you've always done
and be any better tomorrow than you are today. You

don't need to wait until you are critically ill to change your lifestyle. Take charge. Make changes. Make better choices in the six essential areas of life.

WELLNESS PRINCIPLE: **Choose health as your main course from the menu of life.**

CHAPTER 11

SAMPLE MENUS

PUTTING IT ALL TOGETHER

Now you know why the food you eat plays such an important part in your health. We've done the class work, now comes the practical application.

A few words about the menus in this chapter.

The first menu, shown with a shaded background, is a sample menu of the typical American diet. It isn't a model for you to follow. It is included for comparison purposes — to show the difference between the typical American diet and the preferred "body-friendly" diet.

The daily menus are designed with two alkalizing meal replacements. Although Alka·Slim™ is designated, any *comparable* alkalizing meal replacement is acceptable. The remaining meal should be eaten in its entirety. "Breakfast" and "Dinner" meals may be eaten any time during the day.

Although your goal is not to be a gram counter, the menus show the gram content for the foods in each meal. This is to help you become familiar with the foods that provide your body with needed nutrition without overloading on calories, protein, fat, or carbohydrates. Where appropriate, "T" indicates a "trace" of a gram. Traces of grams are not included in the total gram count for the day.

Where "juice" is listed in the menus, you can use any 100% pure fruit juice. In designing these meals, apple juice was the juice used. Be sure to use *pure* fruit juice, not "fruit drinks."

Where a choice of foods is indicated, such as honey, maple syrup, or molasses, the grams are given for the food with the highest gram count.

If you currently include meat in your diet more than once a day, use the alkalizing meal replacement only *once* a day for the first week and double the other *food* portions for your other two meals. After the first week, follow the menu plan.

Keep in mind that your body may need to adjust to this new way of eating. You may not feel as well as you like during the first few days of the adjustment period. Hang in there. After your body begins to acclimate to the kinds of foods it should have been getting all along, you should gradually feel better and have more energy. That's what you're working toward — a healthier, happier, more energetic life.

Go for it!

Menu Memo

During the first week of your new, improved eating, use the "Starter Menus." Choose a page for the day, and eat the foods listed on that page. This is not the time for mix and match.

Substitutions should be limited to the salad dressings. "Approved" substitutions, along with the "salad" recipe, are shown on page 193.

After the first week — or when your body begins to become accustomed to the new foods — make your food selections from the "Regular Menus." As you learn more about menu planning, you can design your own.

TYPICAL AMERICAN DIET - CONSERVATIVE

Food	Calories	Protein Gram	Fat Gram	Carbo-hydrate Gram
BREAKFAST				
Eggs, 2 fried	190	12	14	1
Bacon, 3 slices	110	6	9	T
Biscuits, 2; 2 tsp butter	260	4	14	28
LUNCH				
Hamburger, 6 oz	490	40	36	0
Bun, 1	130	4	2	24
Catsup, 2 Tbsp	30	T	T	8
Cheese, 1 slice	160	10	12	4
French fries, 20	320	4	16	20
Cola , 12 oz	160	0	0	41
DINNER				
Steak, 6 oz	480	46	30	0
Potato, baked	220	5	T	51
Salad with dressing	220	2	T	25
Corn, whole kernal, 1 C	165	5	1	41
Bread with butter	270	5	42	14
Coffee	0	0	0	0
Totals	3205	143	176	257
IDEAL	1250	30	10	250

**NOT RECOMMENDED
THIS IS FOR COMPARISON PURPOSES ONLY**

The salads and dressings throughout this program have been based on the following:

The SALADS listed are:

Lettuce, 2 C	20	2	T	4
Tomato, 1 2 3/5" in dia	25	1	T	5
Green pepper, 1	20	1	T	4
Green onions, 6	10	1	T	2
Cucumber, 6 slices	5	T	T	T
TOTAL	**80**	**5**	**T**	**15**

The DRESSINGS listed are:

Vinegar, 4 Tbsp	0	0	0	4
Honey, 1 Tbsp	65	0	0	17
TOTAL	**65**	**0**	**0**	**21**

You may substitute the following				
Lemon juice, 4 Tbsp	15	T	T	4
Maple syrup, 1 Tbsp	61	0	0	16
Molasses, 1 Tbsp	43	0	0	11
Make calculation adjustments !!!				
These are the only substitutions permitted during the STARTER week				

STARTER MENU

Food	Calories	Protein Gram	Fat Gram	Carbo-hydrate Gram
BREAKFAST				
Brown rice, 1 C, moist	230	5	1	50
Honey or maple syrup, 1 Tbsp	65	0	0	17
Peaches, 2 raw	70	2	T	20
Whole wheat toast, 1 slice	70	3	1	13
Butter, 1 ½ tsp	50	T	6	T
Jam, 1 Tbsp	55	T	T	14
SNACK				
Peaches, 2 raw	70	2	T	20
LUNCH				
Alka•Slim™ 2 scoops in 1 C juice	196	7½	1	38
SNACK				
1 hour before or after *either* **Alka•Slim** meal, 3# watermelon, weighed with rind	232	4	3	52
DINNER				
Alka•Slim™ 2 scoops in 1 C juice	196	7½	1	38
Totals	**1234**	**31**	**13**	**262**
IDEAL	**1250**	**30**	**10**	**250**

STARTER MENU				
Food	Calories	Protein Gram	Fat Gram	Carbo-hydrate Gram
BREAKFAST				
Brown rice, 1 C, moist	230	5	1	50
Honey, 2 Tbsp	130	0	0	34
Toast, whole wheat, 2 slices	140	6	2	26
Butter, 1½ tsp	50	T	6	T
Jam, 1 Tbsp	55	T	T	14
Fruit juice, 2 C	230	T	T	58
LUNCH				
Alka•Slim™ 2 scoops in 1 C juice	196	7½	1	38
DINNER				
Alka•Slim™ 2 scoops in 1 C juice	196	7½	1	38
Totals	1227	26	11	258
IDEAL	1250	30	10	250

STARTER MENU				
Food	Calories	Protein Gram	Fat Gram	Carbo-hydrate Gram
BREAKFAST (once per week)				
Oatmeal, 1 C	145	6	2	25
Honey, 2 Tbsp	130	0	0	35
Milk, low fat 2%, 1 C	120	8	5	12
Toast, whole wheat, 1 slice	70	3	1	13
Jam, 1 Tbsp	55	T	T	14
Fruit juice, 1 C	115	T	T	29
LUNCH				
Alka•Slim™ 2 scoops in 1 C juice	196	7½	1	38
Fruit juice, 1 C	115	T	T	29
DINNER				
Alka•Slim™ 2 scoops in 1 C juice	196	7½	1	38
SNACK				
Fruit juice, 1 C	115	T	T	29
Totals	1249	32	10	243
IDEAL	1250	30	10	250

STARTER MENU				
Food	Calories	Protein Gram	Fat Gram	Carbo-hydrate Gram
BREAKFAST - (once per week)				
Fruit juice, 1 C	115	T	T	29
Egg, 1 poached	80	6	6	1
Toast, whole wheat, 2 slices	140	6	2	26
Butter, 1 tsp	35	T	4	T
Jam, 1 Tbsp	55	T	T	14
LUNCH				
Alka•Slim™ 2 scoops in 1 C juice	196	7½	1	38
Fruit juice, 1 C	115	T	T	29
DINNER				
Alka•Slim™ 2 scoops in 1 C juice	196	7½	1	38
Peaches, 2 raw	70	2	T	20
SNACK				
Fruit juice, 1C	115	T	T	29
Totals	1117	29	14	224
IDEAL	1250	30	10	250

STARTER MENU

Food	Calories	Protein Gram	Fat Gram	Carbo-hydrate Gram
BREAKFAST				
Cheerios, Corn Flakes, 1¼ C **OR**	110	2	T	24
Shredded Wheat, ⅔ C *	100	3	1	23
Milk, low fat 2%	120	8	5	12
Toast, whole wheat, 2 slices	140	6	2	26
Sugar, white, 1 Tbsp	45	0	0	12
Jam, 2 Tbsp	110	T	T	28
Fruit juice, 2 C	230	T	T	58
LUNCH				
Alka•Slim™ 2 scoops in 1 C juice	196	7½	1	38
DINNER				
Alka•Slim™ 2 scoops in 1 C juice	196	7½	1	38
* First number used in calculation of totals				
Totals	**1147**	**31**	**9**	**236**
IDEAL	**1250**	**30**	**10**	**250**

STARTER MENU				
Food	Calories	Protein Gram	Fat Gram	Carbo-hydrate Gram
BREAKFAST				
Peaches, 2	70	2	1	20
Pancakes, whole wheat, 2, 4" dia	110	4	4	12
Egg, poached, 1	80	6	6	1
Maple Syrup, 2 Tbsp	122	0	0	32
Fruit juice, 2 C	230	0	0	58
LUNCH				
Alka•Slim™ 2 scoops in 1 C juice	196	7½	1	38
DINNER				
Alka•Slim™ 2 scoops in 1 C juice	196	7½	1	38
Fruit juice, 1 C	115	T	T	29
Totals	**1119**	**27**	**13**	**228**
IDEAL	**1250**	**30**	**10**	**250**

STARTER MENU

Food	Calories	Protein Gram	Fat Gram	Carbo-hydrate Gram
BREAKFAST - (once per week)				
Oatmeal, 1½ C, moist	217	9	3	37
Honey or maple syrup, 2 T	130	0	0	34
Butter, 1½ tsp	50	T	6	T
Toast, whole wheat, 1 slice	70	3	1	13
Jam, 1 Tbsp	55	T	T	14
Fruit juice, 1 C	115	T	T	29
LUNCH				
Alka•Slim™ 2 scoops in 1 C juice	196	7½	1	38
Fruit Juice, 1 C	115	T	T	29
DINNER				
Alka•Slim™ 2 scoops in 1 C juice	196	7½	1	38
Totals	1144	27	12	232
IDEAL:	1250	30	10	250

STARTER MENU				
Food	Calories	Protein Gram	Fat Gram	Carbo- hydrate Gram
BREAKFAST				
Pancakes, whole wheat, 4, 4" in dia	220	8	8	24
Maple syrup, 2 Tbsp	122	0	0	32
Fruit juice, 2 C	230	0	0	58
LUNCH				
Alka•Slim™ 2 scoops in 1 C juice	196	7½	1	38
Banana, 1	105	1	1	27
DINNER				
Alka•Slim™ 2 scoops in 1 C juice	196	7½	1	38
Fruit juice, 1 C	115	0	0	29
Totals	1184	24	11	246
IDEAL	1250	30	10	250

STARTER MENU				
Food	Calories	Protein Gram	Fat Gram	Carbo-hydrate Gram
BREAKFAST				
Alka•Slim™ 2 scoops in 1 C juice	196	7½	1	38
Fruit juice, 1 C	115	T	T	29
LUNCH				
Alka•Slim™ 2 scoops in 1 C juice	196	7½	1	38
Fruit juice, 1 C	115	T	T	29
DINNER				
Cauliflower, 2 C, cooked from raw	60	4	T	12
Sweet corn, 1 5" ear	85	3	1	19
Butter, 1½ tsp	50	T	6	T
Summer squash, 1 C	35	2	1	8
Applesauce, unsweetened, 2 C	210	T	T	56
Salad, 2 C	80	5	T	15
Dressing	65	0	0	21
Peaches, 2 raw	70	2	T	20
Totals	**1277**	**31**	**10**	**285**
IDEAL	**1250**	**30**	**10**	**250**

STARTER MENU

Food	Calories	Protein Gram	Fat Gram	Carbo-hydrate Gram
BREAKFAST				
Alka•Slim™ 2 scoops in 1 C juice	196	7½	1	38
LUNCH				
Alka•Slim™ 2 scoops in 1 C juice	196	7½	1	38
DINNER				
White potato, baked with skin, ½ lb	220	5	T	51
Butter, 1½ tsp	50	T	6	T
Cabbage, cooked, 2 C	60	2	T	14
Leaf lettuce, shredded, 2 C	20	2	T	4
Dressing	65	0	0	21
Carrots, cooked from raw, 1 C	70	2	T	16
Asparagus, 1 C	45	5	1	8
SNACK:				
Fruit juice, 1 C	115	T	T	29
Totals	1037	31	9	219
IDEAL	1250	30	10	250

STARTER MENU

Food	Calories	Protein Gram	Fat Gram	Carbo-hydrate Gram
BREAKFAST				
Alka•Slim™ 2 scoops in 1 C juice	196	7½	1	38
LUNCH				
Alka•Slim™ 2 scoops in 1 C juice	196	7½	1	38
DINNER				
Green beans, 1 C, canned	25	2	T	6
Butter, 1½ tsp	50	T	6	T
Butter leaf lettuce	20	2	T	4
Tomato, 1 2 3/5"	25	1	T	5
Green pepper, 1 whole	20	1	T	4
Green onions, 6	10	1	T	2
Cucumber, 6 slices w/ peel, 2⅛" dia	5	T	T	T
Dressing	65	0	0	21
Applesauce, 2 C, sweetened	390	T	T	102
Lima beans, ½ C, canned	130	8	T	25
Totals	1132	30	8	102
IDEAL	1250	30	10	250

STARTER MENU				
Food	Calories	Protein Gram	Fat Gram	Carbo-hydrate Gram
BREAKFAST				
Alka•Slim™ 2 scoops in 1 C juice	196	7½	1	38
Juice, 1 C	115	T	T	29
LUNCH				
Alka•Slim™ 2 scoops in 1 C juice	196	7½	1	38
Banana, 2	210	2	2	54
DINNER				
Peas. ½ C, cooked from frozen	62	4	T	11
Sweet potato, baked in skin, 6 oz	115	2	T	28
Butter, 1 tsp	35	T	4	T
Salad	80	5	T	15
Dressing	65	0	0	21
Totals	1074	28	8	234
IDEAL	1250	30	10	250

STARTER MENU

Food	Calories	Protein Gram	Fat Gram	Carbo-hydrate Gram
BREAKFAST				
Alka•Slim™ 2 scoops in 1 C juice	196	7½	1	38
Fruit juice, 1 C	115	T	T	29
LUNCH				
Alka•Slim™ 2 scoops in 1 C juice	196	7½	1	38
DINNER				
Sweet potato, baked in skin , 12 oz	230	4	T	56
Butter, 1½ tsp	50	T	6	T
Salad	80	5	T	15
Dressing	65	T	T	21
Green beans, 2 C, canned	50	4	T	12
Applesauce, unsweetened, 2 C	210	T	T	56
Tomatoes, cherry, 5	25	1	T	5
Totals	1217	29	8	270
IDEAL	1250	30	10	250

STARTER MENU				
Food	Calories	Protein Gram	Fat Gram	Carbo-hydrate Gram
BREAKFAST				
Alka•Slim™ 2 scoops in 1 C juice	196	7½	1	38
Juice, 1 C, (or with dinner)	115	T	T	29
LUNCH				
Alka•Slim™ 2 scoops in 1 C juice	196	7½	1	38
DINNER				
Sweet corn, 5" ears, 2	170	6	2	38
Salad	80	5	T	15
Dressing	65	T	T	21
Green beans, canned, 1 C	25	2	T	6
Carrots, 1 C, cooked from fresh	70	2	T	16
Butter, 1½ tsp	50	T	6	T
Summer squash, 1 C	35	2	1	8
Applesauce, unsweetened, 2 C	210	T	T	56
Totals:	**1212**	**32**	**11**	**265**
IDEAL	**1250**	**30**	**10**	**250**

STARTER MENU				
Food	Calories	Protein Gram	Fat Gram	Carbo-hydrate Gram
BREAKFAST				
Alka•Slim™ 2 scoops in 1 C juice	196	7½	1	38
LUNCH				
Alka•Slim™ 2 scoops in 1 C juice	196	7½	1	38
DINNER				
White potato, baked with skin , ½ lb	220	5	T	51
Butter, 1½ tsp	50	T	6	T
Salad	80	5	T	15
Dressing	65	0	0	21
Tomato, 2 3/5" dia	25	1	T	5
Green beans, 1 C, canned	25	2	T	6
Carrots, 1 C, cooked from raw	70	2	T	16
SNACK				
Banana, 1	105	1	1	27
Blueberries, 1 C, fresh	80	1	1	20
Fruit juice, 1 C	115	T	T	29
Totals	**1227**	**37**	**10**	**266**
IDEAL	**1250**	**30**	**10**	**250**

REGULAR MENU WINTER				
Food	Calories	Protein Gram	Fat Gram	Carbo- hydrate Gram
BREAKFAST				
Alka•Slim™ 2 scoops in 1 C juice	196	7½	1	38
Fruit juice, 1 C, (or with lunch)	115	T	T	29
LUNCH				
Alka•Slim™ 2 scoops in 1 C juice	196	7½	1	38
DINNER				
Sweet potato, 12 oz, baked in skin	230	4	T	56
Butter, 1½ tsp	50	T	6	T
Lettuce, butter leaf, 1 head	20	2	T	4
Tomato, ½	12	½	T	3
Green beans, 2 C	50	4	T	12
Pepper, green or red	20	1	T	4
Green onions, 6	10	1	T	2
Cucumber, 6 slices w/ peel, 2⅛" dia	5	T	T	1
Dressing	65	0	0	21
Applesauce, unsweetened, 2 C	210	T	T	56
Totals	**1179**	**27½**	**8**	**264**
IDEAL	**1250**	**30**	**10**	**250**

REGULAR MENU				
Food	Calories	Protein Gram	Fat Gram	Carbo-hydrate Gram
BREAKFAST				
Oatmeal, 1½ C	217	9	3	37
Maple syrup, 1 Tbsp	61	0	0	16
Toast, Whole wheat, 1 slice	70	3	1	13
Peaches, 2 raw	70	2	T	20
Butter, 1 tsp	35	T	4	T
LUNCH				
Alka•Slim™ 2 scoops in 1 C juice	196	7½	1	38
Raspberries, 1 C, fresh	60	1	1	14
Banana, 1	105	1	1	27
DINNER				
Alka•Slim™ 2 scoops in 1 C juice	196	7½	1	38
Peaches, 2 raw	70	2	T	20
Totals	**1080**	**33**	**12**	**223**
IDEAL	**1250**	**30**	**10**	**250**

REGULAR MENU WINTER

Food	Calories	Protein Gram	Fat Gram	Carbo-hydrate Gram
BREAKFAST				
Egg, 1 boiled	80	6	6	1
Potato, 4 oz, boiled and cut, browned	110	2½	T	27
Butter to brown potato, 1 tsp	35	T	4	T
LUNCH				
Alka•Slim™ 2 scoops in 1 C juice	196	7½	1	38
Juice, 1 C	115	T	T	29
Banana, 1	105	1	1	27
DINNER				
Alka•Slim™ 2 scoops in 1 C juice	196	7½	1	38
Peaches, canned, no sugar, 2 C	220	4	0	58
Yogurt, fruit flavored, 8 oz	230	10	2	43
Totals	1287	38½	15	261
IDEAL	1250	30	10	250

REGULAR MENU WINTER				
Food	Calories	Protein Gram	Fat Gram	Carbo-hydrate Gram
BREAKFAST				
Alka•Slim™ 2 scoops in 1 C juice	196	7½	1	38
Banana, 1	105	1	1	27
LUNCH				
Alka•Slim™ 2 scoops in 1 C juice	196	7½	1	38
Banana, 1	105	1	1	27
SNACK				
Oranges, 2	120	2	T	30
DINNER				
Beans, from dried, any kind, 1 C	230	15	1	45
Carrots, from frozen, 1 C	55	2	T	12
Bread, whole wheat, 1 slice	70	3	1	13
Butter, 1½ tsp	50	0	6	
Salad	80	5	T	15
Dressing	65	0	0	21
Totals	**1272**	**44**	**12**	**266**
IDEAL	**1250**	**30**	**10**	**250**

REGULAR MENU WINTER				
Food	Calories	Protein Gram	Fat Gram	Carbo-hydrate Gram
BREAKFAST				
Alka•Slim™ 2 scoops in 1 C juice	196	7½	1	38
Peaches, canned, no sugar, 1 C	110	2	0	29
LUNCH				
Alka•Slim™ 2 scoops in 1 C juice	196	7½	1	38
DINNER				
Mixed vegetables, 1 C	105	5	T	24
White potato, ½ lb, baked with skin	220	5	T	51
Butter, 1½ tsp	50	T	6	T
Applesauce, sweetened, 1 C	195	T	T	51
Salad	80	5	T	15
Dressing	65	0	0	21
Winter squash	80	2	1	18
Totals	**1297**	**34**	**9**	**285**
IDEAL	**1250**	**30**	**10**	**250**

REGULAR MENU WINTER

Food	Calories	Protein Gram	Fat Gram	Carbo-hydrate Gram
BREAKFAST				
Alka•Slim™ 2 scoops in 1 C juice	196	7½	1	38
Oranges, 2	120	2	T	30
LUNCH				
Alka•Slim™ 2 scoops in 1 C juice	196	7½	1	38
DINNER				
White Potato, ½ lb, baked in skin	220	5	T	51
Gravy: Beef bouillon, 1 cube Water, 1 C	15	1	1	1
Flour, to thicken, 2 Tbsp	50	2	T	11
Cabbage, cooked, 1 C	30	1	T	7
Carrots, cooked from raw, 1 C	70	2	T	16
Salad	80	5	T	15
Dressing	65	0	0	21
Totals	1042	33	3	228
IDEAL	1250	30	10	250

REGULAR MENU WINTER

Food	Calories	Protein Gram	Fat Gram	Carbo-hydrate Gram
BREAKFAST				
Alka•Slim™ 2 scoops in 1 C juice	196	7½	1	38
Peach, 1, canned, no sugar	110	2	T	30
LUNCH				
Alka•Slim™ 2 scoops in 1 C juice	196	7½	1	38
Peach, 1, canned, no sugar	110	2	T	30
DINNER				
Vegetable soup:				
Bouillon,beef, 1 cube in 1 C water	6	1	1	1
Mixed vegetables, frozen, 2 C	210	10	T	48
Onion, ¼ C, chopped	14	½	0	3
Water chestnuts, ½ C, canned	35	T	T	9
Bread, whole wheat, 2 slices	140	6	2	26
Butter, 1½ tsp	50	T	6	T
Dressing	65	0	0	21
Salad	80	5	T	15
Totals	**1212**	**41½**	**11**	**259**
IDEAL	**1250**	**30**	**10**	**250**

REGULAR MENU WINTER				
Food	Calories	Protein Gram	Fat Gram	Carbo-hydrate Gram
BREAKFAST				
Alka•Slim™ 2 scoops in 1 C juice	196	7½	1	38
Banana, 1	105	1	1	27
LUNCH				
Alka•Slim™ 2 scoops in 1 C juice	196	7½	1	38
Banana, 1	105	1	1	27
DINNER				
Brown rice, 1 C, moist	230	5	1	50
Peas, cooked from frozen, 1 C	125	8	T	23
Winter squash, 1 C, fresh	80	2	1	18
Butter, 1 tsp	50	T	6	T
Salad	80	5	T	15
Dressing	65	0	0	21
Totals	**1232**	**37**	**12**	**257**
IDEAL	**1250**	**30**	**10**	**250**

REGULAR MENU WINTER				
Food	Calories	Protein Gram	Fat Gram	Carbo-hydrate Gram
BREAKFAST				
Alka•Slim™ 2 scoops in 1 C juice	196	7½	1	38
Banana, 1	105	1	1	27
LUNCH				
Alka•Slim™ 2 scoops in 1 C juice	196	7½	1	38
DINNER				
Carrots, 1 C, cooked from raw	70	2	T	16
Peas, 1 C, canned	125	8	T	16
Sweet potato, 1 6"x2", baked in skin	115	2	T	23
Bread, whole wheat, 1 slice	70	3	1	13
Butter, 2 1"x1"x⅓" pats	70	T	8	T
Applesauce, sweetened, 1 C	195	T	T	51
Salad	100	6	T	16
Dressing	65	0	0	21
Totals	**1307**	**37**	**12**	**259**
IDEAL	**1250**	**30**	**10**	**250**

REGULAR MENU				
Food	Calories	Protein Gram	Fat Gram	Carbo-hydrate Gram
BREAKFAST				
Alka•Slim™ 2 scoops in 1 C juice	196	7½	1	38
Peaches, 2, raw	70	2	T	20
LUNCH				
Alka•Slim™ 2 scoops in 1 C juice	196	7½	1	38
Banana,1 ; Pears, Bartlett, 2 raw	305	3	3	62
DINNER - (one time per week)				
Stir Fry: Oil , 1 Tbsp	125	0	14	0
Mung bean sprouts, 1 C, fresh	30	3	T	5
Summer squash, 1 C, fresh	35	2	1	8
Green papper, 1 ; sliced onion, ½ C	40	1	T	8
Water chestnuts, canned, 1 C	70	1	T	17
Cauliflower, 1 C, fresh	25	2	T	5
Bamboo shoots, canned, ½ C	12	1	T	4
Soy sauce, 2 tsp	6	1	1	2
Tomato, 1 in wedges, add at last	25	1	T	5
Totals	**1135**	**32**	**21**	**212**
IDEAL	**1250**	**30**	**10**	**250**

REGULAR MENU				
Food	Calories	Protein Gram	Fat Gram	Carbo-hydrate Gram
BREAKFAST				
Alka•Slim™ 2 scoops in 1 C juice	196	7½	1	38
Fruit juice, 1 C	115	T	T	29
LUNCH				
Alka•Slim™ 2 scoops in 1 C juice	196	7½	1	38
DINNER (one time per week)				
Fettucine with Asparagus				
Fettucine, egg, 1 C	200	7	2	37
Olive Oil, 1 Tbsp	125	0	14	0
Garlic, ½ clove, basil or cilantro				
Asparagus, 4 spears	10	1	T	2
Tomatoes, cherry, 5	25	1	T	5
Salad	80	5	T	15
Dressing	65	0	0	21
Peach, 1	35	1	T	10
Carrots, 1 C	70	2	T	12
Totals	**1117**	**32**	**18**	**207**
IDEAL	**1250**	**30**	**10**	**250**

REGULAR MENU (once per week)				
Food	Calories	Protein Gram	Fat Gram	Carbo-hydrate Gram
BREAKFAST				
Alka•Slim™ 2 scoops in 1 C juice	196	7½	1	38
Fruit juice, 1 C	115	T	T	29
LUNCH				
Alka•Slim™ 2 scoops in 1 C juice	196	7½	1	38
DINNER - Black Beaen Chili				
Saute in sesame see oil, 1 Tbsp	125	0	14	0
Yellow onion, diced, ½ C	30	2	T	13
Celery / carrots, ½ C each, diced	45	1	T	12
Cover, simmer 20 min				
Add: Black beans, canned, 1 C	75	5	T	14
Cumin, chili powser, salt, black pepper, chili pepper seeds, tamari, jalapeno juice (drops), garlic, to taste				
Tomatoes, 2, cut	50	2	T	10
Pepper, ½ green; ½ yellow	20	T	T	4
Green beans, 1 C, canned	25	2	T	6
Potato, boiled, ½ lb	220	5	T	51
Totals	**1097**	**32**	**16**	**215**
IDEAL	**1250**	**30**	**10**	**250**

MAINTENANCE MENU			
Food	Calories	Protein Gram	Fat Gram	Carbo-hydrate Gram
BREAKFAST				
Brown rice, moist, 2 C	230	5	1	50
Honey, 2 Tbsp	130	0	0	34
Toast, whole wheat, 2 slices	140	6	2	26
Butter, 1 tsp	50	T	6	T
Jam, 1 Tbsp	55	T	T	14
Fruit juice, 2 C	230	T	T	58
LUNCH				
Alka•Slim™ 2 scoops in 1 C juice	196	7½	1	38
DINNER				
Sweet potato, baked in skin, 6 oz	115	2	T	28
Cauliflower, cooked from raw, 1 C	30	2	T	6
English muffin, 1	140	5	1	27
Totals	**1316**	**27½**	**11**	**281**
IDEAL	**1250**	**30**	**10**	**250**

MAINTENANCE MENU

Food	Calories	Protein Gram	Fat Gram	Carbo-hydrate Gram
BREAKFAST				
Alka•Slim™ 2 scoops in 1 C juice	196	7½	1	38
Banana, 2	210	2	2	54
LUNCH				
Brown rice, 1 C, moist	230	5	1	50
Peaches, canned, juice pack, 1 C	110	2	T	29
Bread, whole wheat, 1 slice	70	3	1	13
Apple juice, 1 C	115	T	T	29
DINNER				
Sweet potato, 6 oz, baked in skin	115	2	T	28
Butter, 1½ tsp	50	T	6	T
Carrots, cooked from frozen, 1 C	55	2	T	12
Totals	1151	23½	11	253
IDEAL	1250	30	10	250

MAINTENANCE MENU				
Food	Calories	Protein Gram	Fat Gram	Carbo-hydrate Gram
BREAKFAST				
Alka•Slim™ 2 scoops in 1 C juice	196	7½	1	38
Orange juice, 1 C	110	. 2	T	27
LUNCH				
Peaches, canned, no sugar, ½ C	55	1	0	12
Bananas, 2	210	2	2	54
Apple juice, 1 C	115	T	T	29
DINNER				
Salmon, 2 oz pink, boneless, water pack	90	14	3	0
Green beans, canned, 1 C	25	2	T	6
Applesauce, sweetened, 1 C	195	T	T	51
Bread, whole wheat, 1 slice	70	3	1	13
Butter, 1 tsp	35	T	6	T
Salad	80	5	T	16
Dressing	65	T	T	21
Totals	**1246**	**36½**	**13**	**267**
IDEAL	**1250**	**30**	**10**	**250**

MAINTENANCE MENU				
Food	Calories	Protein Gram	Fat Gram	Carbo-hydrate Gram
BREAKFAST				
Alka•Slim™ 2 scoops in 1 C juice	196	7½	1	38
Banana, 1	105	1	1	27
LUNCH				
Roast beef, 2.8 oz lean, round	175	25	8	0
Pineapple, 1 slice, juice pack	35	T	T	9
Carrots, 1 C, cooked from frozen	55	2	T	12
Cauliflower, cooked from raw	30	2	T	6
Applesauce, 2 C, sweetened	390	T	T	102
DINNER				
Salad	80	5	T	15
Vinegar/honey dressing	65	0	0	21
Totals	1131	42½	10	230
IDEAL	1250	30	10	250

MAINTENANCE MENU				
Food	Calories	Protein Gram	Fat Gram	Carbo-hydrate Gram
BREAKFAST				
Alka•Slim™ 2 scoops in 1 C juice	196	7½	1	38
Fruit juice, 1 C	115	T	T	29
LUNCH				
Alka•Slim™ 2 scoops in 1 C juice	196	7½	1	38
Fruit juice, 1 C	115	T	T	29
DINNER				
Salad	80	5	T	16
Dressing	65	T	T	21
Steam celery, onion, 1 C each	75	3	T	16
Add: Tomato, canned or fresh, 1 C	50	2	1	10
Basil, parsley, garlic, salt, 1 tsp each				
Cabbage, chunked, 1 C	15	1	T	4
Beef boullion, 1 cube	15	1	1	1
Bean with bacon soup, 1 C	170	8	6	23
Zucchini, chunked, 1 C	35	2	1	8
Totals	**1152**	**37**	**11**	**232**
IDEAL	**1250**	**30**	**10**	**250**

ENDNOTES

1. Hegsted, D.M. Calcium and Osteoporosis. J. Nutr., 116, p. 2316, 1986.

2. Joslyn, Maynard A., Ed. *Methods in Food Analysis: Physical, Chemical, and Instrumental Methods of Analysis*, 2nd ed. New York: Academic Press, 1970, p. 123.

3. Ibid.

4. Robinson, C. H. *Normal and Therapeutic Nutrition*, 13th ed. New York: Macmillan Co., 1967, p. 131.

APPENDIX

Table A–5. Amino Acid Content of Selected Foods*

(per 100 grams food, edible portion)

Food	Protein gm	Trypto-phan gm	Threo-nine gm	Iso-leucine gm	Leucine gm	Lysine gm	Sulfur Containing Methionine gm	Cystine gm	Phenyl-alanine gm	Tyrosine gm	Valine gm	Arginine gm	Histidine gm
Milk													
Cow:													
Fluid, whole and nonfat	3.5	0.049	0.161	0.223	0.344	0.272	0.086	0.031	0.170	0.178	0.240	0.128	0.092
Canned:													
Evaporated, unsweetened	7.0	.099	.323	.447	.688	.545	.171	.063	.340	.357	.481	.256	.185
Condensed, sweetened	8.1	.114	.374	.518	.796	.631	.198	.072	.393	.413	.557	.296	.214
Dried													
Whole	25.8	.364	1.191	1.648	2.535	2.009	.632	.231	1.251	1.316	1.774	.944	.680
Nonfat	35.6	.502	1.641	2.271	3.493	2.768	.870	.318	1.724	1.814	2.444	1.300	.937
Goat	3.3	.039	.217	.087	.278	.312	.065	—	.121	—	.139	.174	.068
Human	1.4	.023	.062	.075	.124	.090	.028	.027	.060	.071	.086	.055	.030
Milk Products													
Buttermilk	3.5	.038	.165	.219	.348	.291	.082	.032	.186	.137	.262	.168	.099
Casein	100.0	1.335	4.227	6.550	10.048	8.013	3.084	.382	5.389	5.819	7.393	4.070	3.021
Cheese													
Blue mold	21.5	.293	.799	1.449	2.096	1.577	.559	.121	1.153	1.028	1.543	.785	.701
Camembert	17.5	.239	.650	1.179	1.706	1.284	.455	.099	.938	.837	1.256	.639	.571
Cheddar	25.0	.341	.929	1.685	2.437	1.834	.650	.141	1.340	1.195	1.794	.913	.815
Cheddar processed	23.2	.316	.862	1.563	2.262	1.702	.604	.131	1.244	1.109	1.665	.847	.756
Cottage	17.0	.179	.794	.989	1.826	1.428	.469	.147	.917	.917	.978	.802	.549
Cream cheese	9.0	.080	.408	.519	.923	.721	.229	.085	.547	.408	.538	.313	.278

* Items selected from Amino Acid Content of Foods, by M. L. Orr and B. K. Watt, Home Economics Research Rep. No. 4, Agricultural Research Service, U.S. Department of Agriculture, Washington, 1957.

Table A–5. Amino Acid Content of Selected Foods (Continued)

(per 100 grams food, edible portion)

Food	Protein gm	Tryptophan gm	Threonine gm	Isoleucine gm	Leucine gm	Lysine gm	Sulfur Containing Methionine gm	Cystine gm	Phenylalanine gm	Tyrosine gm	Valine gm	Arginine gm	Histidine gm
Swiss	27.5	0.375	1.021	1.853	2.681	2.017	0.715	0.155	1.474	1.315	1.974	1.004	0.896
Swiss processed	26.4	.360	.981	1.779	2.574	1.937	.687	.149	1.415	1.262	1.895	.964	.861
Eggs													
Whole	12.8	.211	.637	.850	1.126	.819	.401	.299	.739	.551	.950	.840	.307
Whites	10.8	.164	.477	.698	.950	.648	.420	.263	.689	.449	.842	.634	.233
·Yolks	16.3	.235	.827	.996	1.372	1.074	.417	.274	.717	.756	1.121	1.132	.368
Meat and poultry													
Beef cuts, medium fat													
Chuck	18.6	.217	.821	.973	1.524	1.625	.461	.235	.765	.631	1.033	1.199	.646
Hamburger	16.0	.187	.707	.837	1.311	1.398	.397	.202	.658	.543	.888	1.032	.556
Porterhouse	16.4	.192	.724	.858	1.343	1.433	.407	.207	.674	.556	.911	1.057	.569
Rib roast	17.4	.203	.768	.910	1.425	1.520	.432	.220	.715	.590	.966	1.122	.604
Round	19.5	.228	.861	1.020	1.597	1.704	.484	.246	.802	.661	1.083	1.257	.677
Rump	16.2	.189	.715	.848	1.327	1.415	.402	.205	.666	.550	.899	1.045	.562
Sirloin	17.3	.202	.764	.905	1.417	1.511	.429	.219	.711	.587	.960	1.116	.601
Beef, dried or chipped	34.3	.401	1.515	1.795	2.810	2.996	.851	.434	1.410	1.163	1.904	2.212	1.191
Lamb cuts, medium fat													
Leg	18.0	.233	.824	.933	1.394	1.457	.432	.236	.732	.625	.887	1.172	.501
Rib	14.9	.193	.682	.772	1.154	1.206	.358	.195	.606	.517	.734	.970	.415
Shoulder	15.6	.202	.714	.809	1.208	1.263	.374	.205	.634	.542	.769	1.016	.434
Pork cuts, medium fat, fresh													
Ham	15.2	.197	.705	.781	1.119	1.248	.379	.178	.598	.542	.790	.931	.525
Loin	16.4	.213	.761	.842	1.207	1.346	.409	.192	.646	.585	.853	1.005	.567
Miscellaneous lean cuts	14.5	.188	.673	.745	1.067	1.190	.362	.169	.571	.517	.754	.889	.501

+ Essential Amino Acids

Food													
Pork, cured													
Bacon, medium fat	9.1	0.095	0.306	0.399	0.728	0.587	0.141	0.106	0.434	0.234	0.434	0.622	0.246
Fat back or salt pork	3.9	.006	.141	.110	.367	.317	.055	.043	.157	.052	.168	.379	.035
Ham	16.9	.162	.692	.841	1.306	1.420	.411	.273	.646	.652	.879	1.068	.544
Luncheon meat													
Boiled ham	22.8	.219	.934	1.135	1.762	1.915	.554	.368	.872	.879	1.186	1.441	.733
Canned, spiced	14.9	.143	.610	.741	1.151	1.252	.362	.241	.570	.575	.775	.942	.479
Veal cuts, medium fat													
Round	19.5	.256	.846	1.030	1.429	1.629	.446	.231	.792	.702	1.008	1.270	.627
Shoulder	19.4	.255	.841	1.024	1.422	1.620	.444	.230	.788	.698	1.003	1.263	.624
Stew meat	18.3	.240	.793	.966	1.341	1.528	.419	.217	.744	.659	.946	1.192	.589
Chicken, flesh only													
Broilers or fryers	20.6	.250	.877	1.088	1.490	1.810	.537	.277	.811	.725	1.012	1.302	.593
Hens	21.3	.259	.907	1.125	1.540	1.871	.556	.286	.838	.750	1.046	1.346	.613
Fish and shellfish													
Blue fish	20.5	.203	.889	1.040	1.548	1.797	.597	.276	.761	.554	1.092	1.155	—
Cod, fresh	16.5	.164	.715	.837	1.246	1.447	.480	.222	.612	.446	.879	.929	—
dried	81.8	.811	3.547	4.149	6.178	7.172	2.382	1.099	3.036	2.212	4.358	4.607	—
Flounder	14.9	.148	.646	.756	1.125	1.306	.434	.200	.553	.403	.794	.839	—
Haddock	18.2	.181	.789	.923	1.374	1.596	.530	.245	.676	.492	.970	1.025	—
Halibut	18.6	.185	.806	.943	1.405	1.631	.542	.250	.690	.503	.991	1.048	—
Herring, Atlantic	18.3	.182	.793	.928	1.382	1.605	.533	.246	.679	.495	.975	1.031	—
Mackerel, raw, common Atlantic	18.7	.186	.811	.948	1.412	1.640	.545	.251	.694	.506	.996	1.053	—
Salmon, raw, Pacific	17.4	.173	.754	.883	1.314	1.526	.507	.234	.646	.470	.927	.980	—
canned, red, solids and liquid	20.2	.200	.876	1.025	1.526	1.771	.588	.271	.750	.546	1.076	1.138	—
Sardines, canned, solids and liquid, Atlantic	21.1	.209	.915	1.070	1.593	1.850	.614	.284	.783	.571	1.124	1.188	—
Shrimp, canned, solids and liquid	18.7	.186	.811	.948	1.412	1.640	.545	.251	.694	.506	.996	1.053	—

Table A–5. Amino Acid Content of Selected Foods (Continued)

(per 100 grams food, edible portion)

+ Essential Amino Acids

Food	Protein gm	Trypto-phan gm	Threo-nine gm	Iso-leucine gm	Leucine gm	Lysine gm	Sulfur Containing Methionine gm	Cystine gm	Phenyl-alanine gm	Tyrosine gm	Valine gm	Arginine gm	Histidine gm
Products from meat, poultry and fish													
Fish flour	76.0	0.754	4.378	4.232	6.189	7.381	2.019	—	2.845	—	3.916	5.204	1.289
Gelatin	85.6	.006	1.912	1.357	2.930	4.226	.787	.077	2.036	.401	2.421	7.866	.771
Liver, beef or pork	19.7	.296	.936	1.031	1.819	1.475	.463	.243	.993	.738	1.239	1.201	.523
Sausage													
Bologna	14.8	.126	.606	.718	1.061	1.191	.313	.185	.540	.481	.744	1.028	.398
Frankfurters	14.2	.120	.582	.688	1.018	1.143	.300	.177	.518	.461	.713	.986	.382
Liverwurst	16.7	.187	.724	.818	1.400	1.301	.347	.203	.759	.510	1.037	1.034	.497
Pork, links or bulk, raw	10.8	.092	.442	.524	.774	.869	.228	.135	.394	.351	.543	.750	.290
Pork, bulk, canned	15.4	.131	.631	.747	1.104	1.239	.325	.192	.562	.500	.774	1.069	.414
Salami	23.9	.203	.979	1.159	1.713	1.923	.505	.298	.872	.776	1.201	1.660	.642
Tongue, beef	16.4	.197	.708	.792	1.286	1.364	.357	.207	.661	.548	.840	1.065	.412
Legumes													
Beans													
Red kidney													
raw	23.1	.214	1.002	1.312	1.985	1.715	.233	.229	1.275	.891	1.401	1.390	.658
canned, solids and liquid	5.7	.053	.247	.324	.490	.423	.057	.057	.315	.220	.346	.343	.162
Other common beans including navy, pea-bean, white marrow:													
raw	21.4	.199	.928	1.216	1.839	1.589	.216	.212	1.181	.825	1.298	1.287	.609
baked with pork, canned	5.8	.057	.274	.291	.486	.354	.059	.018	.333	.165	.312	.251	.186

Chickpeas	20.8	0.170	0.739	1.195	1.538	1.434	0.276	0.296	1.012	0.692	1.025	1.551	0.559
Cowpeas	22.9	.220	.901	1.110	1.715	1.491	.352	.297	1.198	.678	1.293	1.473	.692
Lentils, whole	25.0	.216	.896	1.316	1.760	1.528	.180	.204	1.104	.664	1.360	1.908	.548
Lima beans	20.7	.195	.980	1.199	1.722	1.378	.331	.311	1.222	.543	1.298	1.315	.669
Peanuts	26.9	.340	.828	1.266	1.872	1.099	.271	.463	1.557	1.104	1.532	3.296	.749
Peanut flour	51.2	.647	1.575	2.410	3.563	2.091	.516	.881	2.963	2.100	2.916	6.273	1.425
Peanut butter	26.1	.330	.803	1.228	1.816	1.066	.263	.449	1.510	1.071	1.487	3.198	.727
Peas, split	24.5	.259	.945	1.380	2.027	1.795	.294	.318	1.235	.988	1.372	2.164	.670
Soybeans, whole	34.9	.526	1.504	2.504	2.946	2.414	.513	.678	1.889	1.216	2.005	2.763	.911
Soybean flour, flakes and grits													
Low fat	44.7	.673	1.926	2.630	3.773	3.092	.658	.869	2.419	1.558	2.568	3.538	1.166
Full fat	35.9	.541	1.547	2.112	3.030	2.483	.528	.698	1.943	1.251	2.062	2.842	.937
Soybean milk	3.4	.051	.176	.175	.305	.269	.054	.071	.195	.193	.186	.302	.121
Nuts													
Almonds	18.6	.176	.610	.873	1.454	.582	.259	.377	1.146	.618	1.124	2.729	.517
Brazil nuts	14.4	.187	.422	.593	1.129	.443	.941	.504	.617	.483	.823	2.247	.367
Cashews	18.5	.471	.737	1.222	1.522	.792	.353	.527	.946	.712	1.592	2.098	.415
Coconut	3.4	.033	.129	.180	.269	.152	.071	.062	.174	.101	.212	.486	.069
Pecans	9.4	.138	.389	.553	.773	.435	.153	.216	.564	.316	.525	1.185	.273
Walnuts (English or Persian)	15.0	.175	.589	.767	1.228	.441	.306	.320	.767	.583	.974	2.287	.405
Other Seeds													
Cottonseed flour and meal	42.3	.591	1.764	1.884	2.945	2.139	.686	.814	2.610	1.365	2.458	5.603	1.325
Safflower seed meal	42.1	.675	1.462	1.914	2.740	1.525	.731	—	2.605	—	2.446	4.623	.985
Sesame seed	19.3	.331	.707	.951	1.679	.583	.637	.495	1.457	.951	.885	1.992	.441
Meal	33.4	.573	1.223	1.645	2.905	1.008	1.103	.857	2.521	1.645	1.531	3.447	.763
Sunflower meal	39.5	.589	1.565	2.191	2.981	1.491	.760	.797	2.094	1.110	2.325	4.069	1.006
Grains and their products													
Barley	12.8	.160	.433	.545	.889	.433	.184	.257	.661	.466	.643	.659	.239
Bread, white (4% nonfat dry milk, flour basis)	8.5	.091	.282	.429	.668	.225	.142	.200	.465	.243	.435	.340	.192

Table A–5. Amino Acid Content of Selected Foods (Continued)

(per 100 grams food, edible portion)

+ Essential Amino Acids

Food	Protein gm	+ Tryptophan gm	+ Threonine gm	+ Isoleucine gm	+ Leucine gm	+ Lysine gm	Sulfur Containing + Methionine gm	Cystine gm	+ Phenylalanine gm	Tyrosine gm	+ Valine gm	Arginine gm	Histidine gm
Cereal combinations													
Corn and soy grits	18.0	0.161	0.792	0.841	1.656	0.772	0.271	0.311	0.832	0.562	1.054	0.982	0.472
Infant food, precooked, mixed cereals with nonfat dry milk and yeast	19.4	.118	—	—	—	.273	.310	.137	.543	.447	—	.447	.233
Oat-corn-rye mixture, puffed	14.5	.172	.545	.841	1.368	.343	.388	.234	.933	.622	.900	.776	.326
Corn grits	8.7	.053	.347	.402	1.128	.251	.161	.113	.395	.532	.444	.306	.180
Cornmeal, degermed	7.9	.048	.315	.365	1.024	.228	.147	.102	.359	.483	.403	.278	.163
Corn flakes	8.1	.052	.275	.306	1.057	.154	.135	.152	.354	.283	.386	.231	.226
Oatmeal	14.2	.183	.470	.733	1.065	.521	.209	.309	.758	.524	.845	.935	.261
Rice flakes or puffed	5.9	.046	—	—	—	.056	—	.044	.286	.124	—	.137	.137
Rice, white and converted	7.6	.082	.298	.356	.655	.300	.137	.103	.382	.347	.531	.438	.128
Rye flour, medium	11.4	.129	.422	.485	.766	.465	.180	.227	.538	.368	.594	.557	.260
Wheat flour													
Whole grain	13.3	.164	.383	.577	.892	.365	.203	.292	.657	.497	.616	.636	.271
White	10.5	.129	.302	.483	.809	.239	.138	.210	.577	.359	.453	.466	.210
Wheat products													
Bran	12.0	.196	.342	.485	.717	.491	.145	.270	.434	.259	.552	.742	.280
Burghul	12.4	.070	—	—	—	.430	.300	.319	—	—	—	—	—
Farina	10.9	.124	—	—	—	.199	.143	.184	.579	.447	—	.424	.268
Flakes	10.8	.121	.356	.496	.891	.360	.127	.191	.478	.311	.572	.559	.231
Germ	25.2	.265	1.343	1.177	1.708	1.534	.404	.287	.908	.882	1.364	1.825	.687
Macaroni or spaghetti	12.8	.150	.499	.642	.849	.413	.193	.243	.669	.422	.728	.582	.303
Noodles, containing egg solids	12.6	.133	.533	.621	.834	.411	.212	.245	.610	.312	.745	.621	.301
Shredded wheat	10.1	.085	.405	.449	.684	.331	.139	.204	.481	.236	.577	.523	.236

Whole wheat with added germ	12.8	0.136	—	—	—	0.466	—	0.246	0.755	0.481	—	0.742	0.371
Fruit													
Bananas, ripe	1.2	.018	—	—	—	.055	.011	—	—	.031	—	—	—
Dates	2.2	.061	.061	.074	.077	.065	.027	—	.063	—	.094	.049	.049
Grapefruit	0.5	.001	—	—	—	.006	.000	—	—	—	—	—	—
Guavas, common	1.0	.010	—	—	—	.030	.010	—	—	—	—	—	—
Limes	0.8	.003	—	—	—	.015	.002	—	—	—	—	—	—
Mangos	0.7	.014	—	—	—	.093	.008	—	—	—	—	—	—
Muskmelons	0.6	.001	—	—	—	.015	.002	—	—	—	—	—	—
Oranges	0.9	.003	—	—	—	.024	.003	—	—	—	—	—	—
Papayas	0.6	.012	—	—	—	.038	.002	—	—	—	—	—	—
Pineapple	0.4	.005	—	—	—	.009	.001	—	—	—	—	—	—
Vegetables													
Asparagus, raw	2.2	.027	.066	.080	.096	.103	.032	—	.069	—	.106	.123	.036
Beans, snap	2.4	.033	.091	.109	.139	.126	.035	.024	.057	.050	.115	.101	.045
Beet greens	2.0	.024	.076	.084	.129	.108	.034	—	.116	—	.101	.083	.026
Beets	1.6	.014	.034	.051	.055	.086	.006	—	.027	—	.049	.028	.022
Broccoli	3.3	.037	.122	.126	.163	.147	.050	—	.119	—	.170	.192	.063
Brussels sprouts	4.4	.044	.153	.186	.194	.197	.046	—	.148	—	.193	.279	.106
Cabbage	1.4	.011	.039	.040	.057	.066	.013	.028	.030	.030	.043	.105	.025
Carrots	1.2	.010	.043	.046	.065	.052	.010	.029	.042	.020	.056	.041	.017
Cauliflower	2.4	.033	.102	.104	.162	.134	.047	—	.075	.034	.144	.110	.048
Celery	1.3	.012	—	—	—	.021	.015	.006	—	.016	—	—	—
Chard	1.4	.014	.058	.060	.076	.055	.004	—	.046	—	.055	.035	.018
Chicory	1.6	.024	—	.137	.407	.052	.016	.006	—	.040	—	.024	.024
Corn, sweet	3.7	.023	.151	—	.653	.137	.072	.062	.207	.124	.231	.174	.095
Cowpeas	9.4	.099	.353	.465	—	.617	.131	—	.523	—	.513	.615	.310
Cucumbers	0.7	.005	.019	.022	.030	.031	.007	—	.016	—	.024	.053	.001
Eggplant	1.1	.010	.038	.056	.068	.030	.006	.006	.048	—	.065	.037	.019
Kale	3.9	.042	.139	.133	.252	.121	.035	.036	.158	—	.184	.202	.062
Lettuce	1.2	.012	—	—	—	.070	.004	—	—	—	—	—	—

Table A-5. Amino Acid Content of Selected Foods (Continued)

(per 100 grams food, edible portion)

Food	Protein gm	Trypto-phan gm	Threo-nine gm	Iso-leucine gm	Leucine gm	Lysine gm	Sulfur Containing Methionine gm	Cystine gm	Phenyl-alanine gm	Tyrosine gm	Valine gm	Arginine gm	Histidine gm
Lima beans	7.5	0.097	0.338	0.460	0.605	0.474	0.080	0.083	0.389	0.259	0.485	0.454	0.247
Mustard greens	2.3	.037	.060	.075	.062	.111	.024	.035	.074	.121	.108	.167	.041
Onions, mature	1.4	.021	.022	.021	.037	.064	.013	—	.039	.046	.031	.180	.014
Peas	6.7	.056	.245	.308	.418	.316	.054	.073	.257	.163	.274	.595	.109
Peppers	1.2	.009	.050	.046	.046	.051	.016	—	.055	—	.033	.024	.014
Potatoes, raw	2.0	.021	.079	.088	.100	.107	.025	.019	.088	.036	.107	.099	.029
Spinach	2.3	.037	.102	.107	.176	.142	.039	.046	.099	.073	.126	.116	.049
Squash, summer	0.6	.005	.014	.019	.027	.023	.008	—	.016	—	.022	.027	.009
Sweetpotatoes, raw	1.8	.031	.085	.087	.103	.085	.033	.029	.100	.081	.135	.094	.036
Tomatoes	1.0	.009	.033	.029	.041	.042	.007	—	.028	.014	.028	.029	.015
Turnips	1.1	—	—	.020	—	.057	.012	—	.020	.029	—	—	—
Turnip greens	2.9	.045	.125	.107	.207	.129	.052	.045	.146	.105	.149	.167	.051
Miscellaneous food items													
Yeast													
Baker's, compressed	10.6*	.122	.655	.655	1.151	.914	.248	.120	.607	.580	.840	.536	.353
Brewer's, dried	36.9*	.710	2.353	2.398	3.226	3.300	.836	.548	1.902	1.902	2.723	2.250	1.251
Primary, dried													
Saccharomyces cerevisiae	36.9*	.636	2.353	2.708	3.300	3.337	.851	.444	1.813	2.472	2.553	1.931	1.103
Torulopsis utilis	36.9*	.636	2.331	3.323	3.707	3.648	.710	.422	2.361	2.464	2.901	3.337	1.251

+ Essential Amino Acids

* Assumes 4/5 of total nitrogen is protein.

INDEX

RESOURCES

Reverse Osmosis Water Equipment

Essential Water & Air
   Contact: Fred Van Liew
   Telephone: 800-964-4303

Alka*Line Alkalizing Products

Alka*Slim
pH Test Paper
   Morter HealthSystem
   1000 West Poplar
   Rogers, AR 72756
   Telephone: 800-874-1478